MRI for Radiographers

Springer

Berlin
Heidelberg
New York
Barcelona
Budapest
Hong Kong
London
Milan
Paris
Tokyo

Philip T. English and Christine Moore

MRI for Radiographers

With 175 Figures

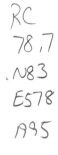

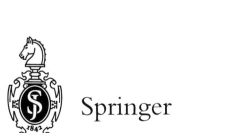 Springer

Philip T. English, DCR
Superintendent Radiographer, Neuroradiology, Newcastle General Hospital, Westgate Road,
Newcastle upon Tyne NE4 6BE, UK

Christine Moore, DCR
Senior Radiographer, Neuroradiology, Newcastle General Hospital,
Westgate Road, Newcastle upon Tyne NE4 6BE, UK

ISBN 3-540-19750 8 Springer-Verlag   Berlin   Heidelberg   New York
ISBN 0-387-19750 8 Springer-Verlag   New York   Berlin   Heidelberg

British Library Cataloguing in Publication Data
   English, Philip T.
   MRI for Radiographers
   I. Title II. Moore, Christine
   616.07548
ISBN 3-540-19750-8

Library of Congress Cataloging-in-Publication Data
English, Philip T., 1961-
   MRI for radiographers/ Philip T. English and Christine Moore.
   Includes bibliographical references and index.
   ISBN 3-540-19750-8 (alk. paper). – ISBN 0-387-19750-8 (alk. paper)
   1. Magnetic resonance imaging.   I. Moore, Christine, 1952-
RC78.7.N83E578 1994
616.07'548--dc20
DNLM/DLC   94-41660
for Library of Congress   CIP

Typeset by EXPO Holdings
Printed and bound by Cambridge University Press
28/3830-543210 Printed on acid-free paper

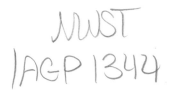

Preface

One of the most important developments in diagnostic imaging over the last decade has been magnetic resonance imaging (MRI). Its ability to differentiate between tissues and give pathological information about diseases has led to earlier treatment, thus increasing the likelihood of recovery. The images produced using this technique give superb anatomical detail in any plane and are obtained without the use of ionising radiation.

The increased use of MRI has presented radiographers with a number of challenges, and because we are no longer dealing with ionising radiation understanding the subject can sometimes be confusing. We hope that this text will help radiographers and student radiographers to further their knowledge and unravel the mysteries of MRI.

Philip T. English
Christine Moore

Contents

1 Basic Principles

History

Magnets were first described by the Romans over 2000 years ago. Over the centuries, as man's understanding of them has increased, so their applications have developed. In the late 1940s two independent groups of scientists led by Felix Bloch (at Stanford) and Edward Purcell (at Harvard) discovered magnetic resonance in liquids and solids respectively. These discoveries led to them being jointly awarded the Nobel Prize in 1952.

Magnetic resonance (MR) was initially used for spectroscopy, and in 1967 MR spectroscopy was used to produce MR signals in a live animal. In the early 1970s Paul Lautebur of the State University of New York produced two-dimensional proton images of a water sample. This work soon led to imaging of other samples, such as lemons and peppers, then live animals and ultimately humans. Magnetic resonance imaging (MRI) was born. Initially the technique was referred to as nuclear magnetic resonance (NMR), but the "nuclear" part of the title had "bad" connotations for the general public and MRI has become the accepted term within the medical profession.

Atomic Theory

Before considering the more complex theory of magnetic resonance we will review a few of the basic principles behind the phenomenon.

All matter is composed of atoms, a different atom corresponding to each chemical element. Under the correct circumstances elements combine to form compounds: for example, sodium and chlorine can combine to form sodium chloride (common salt).

Atoms contain three fundamental particles: electrons, protons and neutrons. The exception is hydrogen, which has a single proton and one orbiting electron. Protons and neutrons are found within the nucleus of the atom and are called collectively "nucleons". The electrons orbit the nucleus at various different energy levels (or shells). Fig. 1.1 is a diagrammatic representation of a neon atom showing how the electrons orbit the nucleus in energy shells.

It can be seen from Table 1.1 that the proton and neutron both have a relative mass of 1 but that the electron has negligible mass. The mass number of an element is the total number of protons and neutrons

Table 1.1. Relative masses and charges of protons, neutrons and electrons

Particle	Relative mass	Relative charge
Proton	1	+1
Neutron	1	0
Electron	1/1837	−1

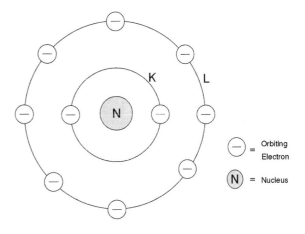

Fig. 1.1. Diagrammatic representation of a neon atom showing the relationships between the nucleus (composed of 10 protons and 10 neutrons) and the electrons. The 10 electrons orbit the nucleus in two energy levels or shells: the K shell and the L shell.

within its nucleus:

Mass number = no. of protons + no. of neutrons

or Mass number = no. of nucleons

It can also be seen from Table 1.1 that protons have a positive charge and electrons have a negative charge. It follows, then, that in order to keep the atom neutral the number of protons must equal the number of electrons.

The atomic number of an element is the number of protons within its nucleus:

Atomic number = no. of protons

The atomic number is also equal to the number of electrons orbiting the nucleus. The atomic number determines the chemical properties of that element.

Magnetic Theory

Atomic Magnetism

The negatively charged electrons orbiting the nucleus spin on their axis in one of two directions: clockwise or anticlockwise. In a non-magnetic element there are the same number of electrons spinning in each direction. In a magnetic element there is an imbalance, with more electrons spinning in one direction than the other. It is this imbalance that creates the potential for magnetism.

An iron atom, for example, has 26 orbiting electrons around its nucleus: 2 electrons in the first (K) shell, 8 electrons in the second (L) shell, 14 electrons in the third (M) shell and 2 electrons in the fourth (N) shell. In the K, L and N shells there are the same number of electrons spinning clockwise as anticlockwise. In the M shell, however, there are 9 electrons spinning in one direction and only 5 spinning in the other, creating an imbalance which gives iron the potential for magnetism.

The magnetic potential of an element can be realised when it is placed in the vicinity of an external magnetic field. The external field encourages the atoms in the element to collect in domains, creating magnetism.

The SI unit for magnetic field strength is the tesla (symbol T). Previously field strength was measured in gauss (1 T = 10 000 gauss).

Nuclear Magnetism

As well as electrons creating magnetism in bulk matter the nuclei of certain atoms are able to create a small magnetic field around themselves. As previously described all atomic nuclei (except for hydrogen) contain both protons and neutrons. When there is an imbalance between the number of protons and the number of neutrons the nucleus will spin upon its axis, and the spinning of the positively charged protons within the nucleus creates a magnetic field. This field is too weak to have any effect on bulk matter and requires very sensitive instruments to detect it. This instrumentation has been developed in the field of magnetic resonance. Table 1.2 lists some of the elements occurring naturally in biological tissue that possess these characteristics.

Seventy-five per cent of the human body consists of water, and therefore it is hydrogen which is the most abundant element in the body. In addition to being a constituent of water, hydrogen is also found in lipids. The hydrogen nucleus is particularly susceptible

Table 1.2. Elements found in the human body that possess magnetic resonance characteristics

Element	Symbol	Nuclear arrangement		Atomic no.
Hydrogen	H	1 proton		1
Carbon	C	6 protons	7 neutrons	13
Fluorine	F	9 protons	10 neutrons	19
Sodium	Na	11 protons	12 neutrons	23
Phosphorus	P	15 protons	16 neutrons	31
Potassium	K	19 protons	20 neutrons	39

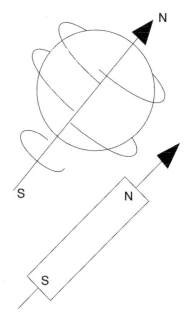

Fig. 1.2. The hydrogen nucleus spinning upon its axis creates a magnetic moment through its axis which is directly comparable to a bar magnet.

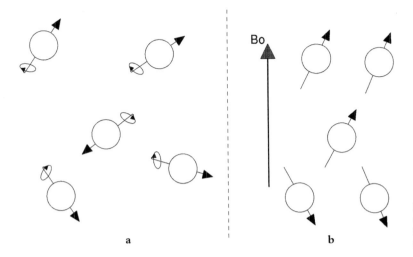

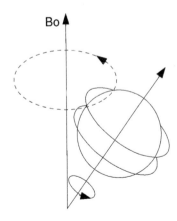

Fig. 1.3a,b The orientation of the magnetic moments of the hydrogen protons in the absence (**a**) and presence (**b**) of an externally applied magnetic field (*Bo*).

to magnetic resonance and its abundance makes it perfect for MRI. Although other elements can be imaged it is hydrogen imaging that will be considered for the rest of the text.

The spinning hydrogen proton can be thought of as a tiny bar magnet with two poles (Fig. 1.2). Each proton generates a magnetic moment, which is a physical vector (represented as an arrow) parallel to its axis of rotation that describes the magnetic field strength and its direction.

In a neutral environment the billions of hydrogen protons in tissues have their magnetic moments randomly orientated (Fig. 1.3a). Placed in a strong magnetic field, such as a magnetic resonance scanner, however, they align themselves in one of two directions: "parallel" or "antiparallel" to the field (Fig. 1.3b), with a slight majority in the parallel direction. The protons which are parallel to the main magnetic field (i.e. aligned towards it) are said to be at a low energy state, whilst those antiparallel to it are said to be at a higher energy state (having sufficient energy to oppose the magnetic field). The actual energy difference between the two states is very small and is dependent upon the field strength.

Thermal energy produced by the various physical and chemical processes within the body causes the two energy states to be almost equally populated. In fact for every 1 million atoms antiparallel to the main field there will be approximately 1 million and six that are parallel! It is this small population difference which gives rise to an overall (or net) magnetisation in the direction of the external main magnetic field (*Bo*) that is detected in MRI. This is known as longitudinal magnetisation.

As shown in Fig. 1.3 the spinning protons do not align themselves exactly with the main magnetic field but more at an angle to it. As the nucleus spins upon

its axis its magnetic moment precesses around the main magnetic field (Fig. 1.4). This precession is similar to the motion of a spinning top, which spins around its axis until the speed of the spin slows, allowing gravity to cause it to precess around the direction of the earth's gravitational field until eventually it falls over. In MR the spinning nucleus precesses in response to the main magnetic field (*Bo*).

The rate of precession of protons in a magnetic field is characteristic for that element; it also depends upon the strength of the magnetic field the element is placed in. This relationship can be expressed as:

$$\omega_0 = \gamma Bo$$

where ω_0 is the angular frequency (precessional or Larmor frequency), γ is the magnetogyric ratio (which depends on the type of nucleus considered) and *Bo* is the magnetic field strength. The equation is known as

Fig. 1.4. Diagrammatic representation of the precession of a hydrogen nucleus around an externally applied main magnetic field (*Bo*).

the Larmor equation after the physicist who first described the phenomenon. What this equation tells us is that if the magnetic field strength changes then so does the rate of precession, i.e. the stronger the magnetic field the faster the rate of precession. For hydrogen the magnetogyric ratio is 4257 Hz (cycles per second) per gauss. Thus at a field strength of 1.5 T (15 000 gauss):

$$\omega_0 = 4257 \times 15\ 000$$

$$= 63\ 855\ 000\ Hz$$

$$= 63.855\ MHz$$

At 1.0 T ω_0 is 42.570 MHz, and at 0.5 T ω_0 is 21.285 MHz.

Resonance

Radiofrequency radiation, or radio waves, are part of the electromagnetic spectrum. Compared with other radiations in the spectrum, however, they are of relatively low energy (Fig. 1.5).

If radiofrequency (RF) radiation at the Larmor frequency is applied to hydrogen nuclei in a magnetic field it induces energy in the hydrogen nuclei sufficient to enable them to oppose the main magnetic field (i.e. to change their alignment from parallel to antiparallel). The exact frequency of the RF radiation is important: if it is not at the Larmor frequency the hydrogen is unable to absorb the energy and nothing happens.

RF radiation, like all electromagnetic radiation, possesses both electrical and magnetic fields (in the same direction but perpendicular to each other). So the RF radiation applied to the hydrogen nuclei can be thought of as a second magnetic field (B1) running perpendicular to the main magnetic field (Bo)

An RF pulse at the Larmor frequency of hydrogen has the following effects: First, it gives sufficient energy to some of the hydrogen nuclei to cause them to align antiparallel to the main magnetic field. Those nuclei now antiparallel cancel out the magnetic effect of the remaining parallel nuclei and this decreases the amount of longitudinal magnetisation. The longitudinal magnetisation may be lost completely, depending on the duration of the RF pulse. What effect does this have on the net magnetisation?

As the amount of longitudinal magnetisation decreases, so there is a gradual increase in the amount of magnetisation in the transverse plane (B1). This magnetisation occurs as a result of the protons which were originally precessing in a random fashion, now precessing "in phase", i.e. in step with one another, causing the summation of their magnetic moments. As all of these moments are precessing around the main magnetic field then this establishes magnetisation in the transverse plane (Fig. 1.6). The longer the RF pulse the more the net magnetisation opposes the main field.

If the RF pulse is short the net magnetisation will rotate away from the main field by an angle known as the flip angle that is proportional to the duration of the RF pulse applied. Flip angles of 90° and 180° are commonly used in MRI.

If hydrogen atoms in a magnetic field are sufficiently excited with RF radiation to produce a 90° flip angle the net magnetisation is transferred to the transverse plane. The magnetic moment will rotate freely (at the Larmor frequency) in the transverse plane, and if a coil of wire is placed adjacent to the hydrogen atoms an alternating current (AC) will be induced into that wire as shown in Fig. 1.7.

Immediately after excitation the maximum signal is induced into the coil, and once the RF pulse stops then the signal begins to decay. This process is known

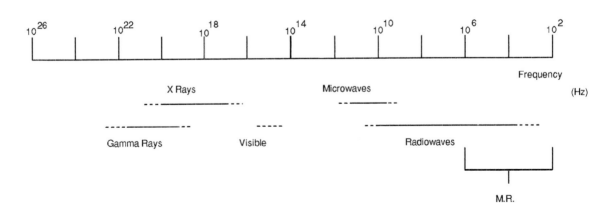

Fig. 1.5.   The spectrum of electromagnetic radiation.

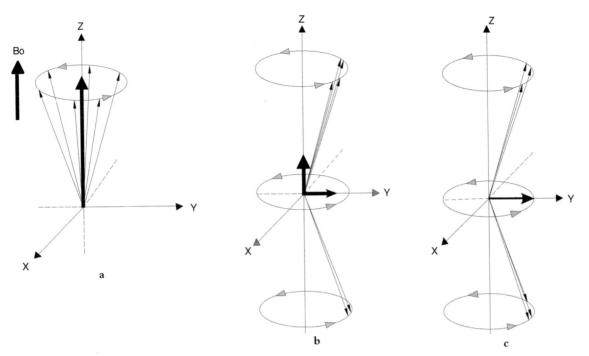

Fig. 1.6 **a** The net magnetisation is in the longitudinal plane (*Z*- axis). There is no magnetisation in the transverse plane (*XY*). **b** After the RF pulse has been applied the longitudinal magnetisation has decreased due to the cancellation effect of the protons parallel and antiparallel to the main magnetic field. Transverse magnetisation is present as the summation of the protons precessing in phase. **c** Longitudinal magnetisation is lost completely when the number of protons antiparallel to the main field is equal to the number that are parallel to it, leaving only the magnetisation in the transverse plane.

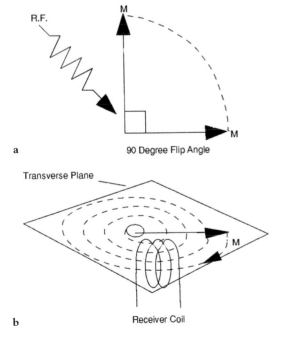

Fig. 1.7 a Following the 90° RF pulse net magnetisation (M) is in the transverse plane. **b** The net magnetisation begins to precess around the longitudinal axis. This results in a current being induced into a receiver coil placed at 90° to the main magnetic field.

as free induction decay. The decay follows an exponential path as the net magnetisation returns to the longitudinal axis, parallel to the main magnetic field (*Bo*). The energy which the nuclei had absorbed is dissipated as heat to the local molecular environment. If signal amplitude is plotted against time an exponential curve is produced that is known as the free induction decay curve (Fig. 1.8). The process by which the signal decays is known as relaxation.

Relaxation

The precise way in which the net magnetisation decays gives important information about the characteristics of the tissues being imaged. There are two features of the relaxation process: (1) transverse (spin–spin) relaxation and (2) longitudinal (spin–lattice) relaxation. These occur simultaneously, but it is easier initially to consider them separately.

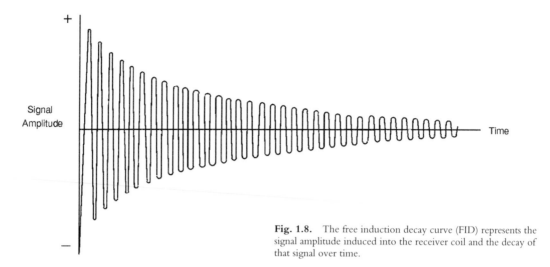

Fig. 1.8. The free induction decay curve (FID) represents the signal amplitude induced into the receiver coil and the decay of that signal over time.

Transverse or Spin–Spin Relaxation

Following a 90° RF pulse the net magnetisation is no longer longitudinal but transverse, that is transverse to the main magnetic field. Therefore just after the 90° pulse the longitudinal magnetisation is zero.

All the hydrogen nuclei which make up that net magnetisation are described as being in phase, or coherent, for a moment, and it is while they are in phase that their combined magnetic moments give the maximum signal. The nuclei begin to precess as soon as the RF pulse is turned off, the rate at which they precess depending on the strength of the magnetic field and the local magnetic environment of the nuclei. In a uniform magnetic field one would expect the nuclei to be precessing at the same speed, that is at the resonant frequency of that nucleus at that magnetic field strength. However, in reality tissue is composed of many different atomic nuclei and electrons possess-

ing their own magnetic moments. These magnetic moments interact with one another and cause local deviations of the magnetic field resulting in some of the hydrogen nuclei precessing at different rates. As time goes on this effect becomes more marked, until eventually there is no longer any net magnetisation in the transverse plane. This is known as loss of phase coherence or dephasing (Fig. 1.9). The time it takes for the net transverse magnetisation to reach equilibrium is known as the time constant T2. Since T2 is an exponential function of time, one T2 interval is the time it takes for 63% of the transverse magnetisation to be lost.

In reality, though, even with modern magnet design it is impossible to achieve a completely homogeneous magnetic field, and this means that the loss of phase coherence occurs quicker than it would if the field were completely homogeneous. The time taken for the loss of the transverse magnetisation under these

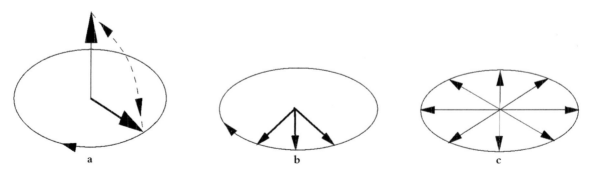

Fig. 1.9. Loss of phase coherence in the transverse plane. **a** Immediately after the 90° pulse the transverse net magnetisation is maximum as all the protons are in phase. **b** Shortly after 90° pulse the protons begin to lose phase. **c** A much longer time after the 90° pulse there is total loss of phase and the result is zero net magnetisation.

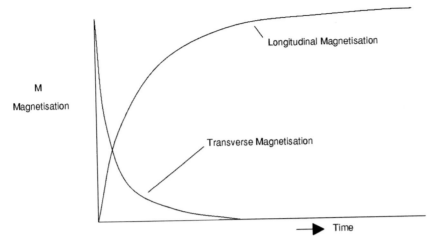

Fig. 1.10. Graph to demonstrate how longitudinal magnetisation increases exponentially with time whereas transverse magnetisation decreases following a 90° RF pulse.

circumstances is known as the time constant T2★. The effect of T2★ can be ruled out by using a special pulse sequence when performing an MR scan.

A pulse sequence is a series of timed RF pulses which are repeated many times during a single acquisition in order to obtain sufficient information for an MR image. The pulse sequence which allows the imaging of T2 is a spin echo sequence, and this will be described along with other pulse sequences in Chapter 3.

Longitudinal or Spin–Lattice Relaxation

The second process which occurs after the excitation of hydrogen nuclei by an RF pulse is the tendency of the nuclei, and therefore of the net magnetisation, to re-align with the main magnetic field.

Immediately following the 90° RF pulse the net magnetisation is in the transverse plane. With time,

though, the energy which the hydrogen nuclei absorbed is lost as heat to the surrounding atoms, and without that extra energy the hydrogen nuclei are unable to oppose the main magnetic field. They therefore re-align with it. The net magnetisation then returns to the longitudinal plane. This relaxation process occurs exponentially.

Longitudinal relaxation has a time constant T1. A tissue's T1 relaxation time is the time taken for the longitudinal magnetisation to reach its equilibrium value. T1 relaxation also occurs in an exponential manner and one T1 interval is the time taken for 63% of the tissue to recover its longitudinal magnetisation.

It is important to realise that longitudinal and transverse relaxation occur together, and that different tissues have different longitudinal and transverse relaxation features. T2 is always shorter than or equal to T1. In fact, comparing the two relaxation processes over time for any given sample gives two exponential curves as shown in Fig. 1.10.

2 Instrumentation

In Chapter 1 we considered the principles behind MRI; we are now going to discuss the hardware required to enable measurements to be made.

The main components of an MRI system are as follows:

1. Magnet
2. Shim coils
3. Gradient coils
4. RF transmitter/receiver coils
5. Computer

The block diagram in Fig. 2.1 shows the layout of these components.

The Magnet

The magnet is the heart of the MRI system. It is the largest and most costly item within the system and there are three primary requirements of it: (1) to produce a magnetic field of a known strength, (2) to produce a homogeneous field and (3) to allow access for patients.

From Chapter 1 we know that the field strength determines the precessional frequency of the protons, so in order to achieve resonance the field strength must be known precisely. The choice of field strength depends on a number of factors such as clinical

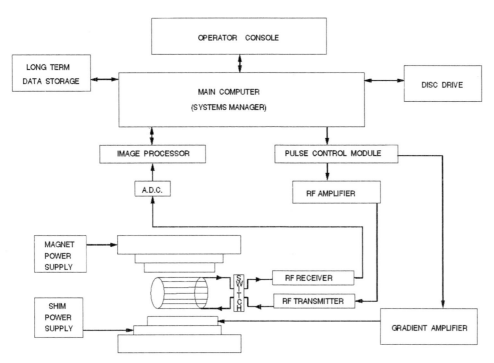

Fig. 2.1. Schematic diagram of the different components of an MRI system. A.D.C, analogue-to-digital converter.

requirements, siting and the finance available, and the final choice is always a compromise between these and other factors. This choice will be discussed in Chapter 10.

The homogeneity of the magnet is measured in parts per million (p.p.m.) and refers to the changes in magnetic field strength within the bore of the magnet. Magnet homogeneity is always quoted by the manufacturer because inhomogeneity of just a few parts per million can lead to noticeable image degradation. Larger inhomogeneity can give rise to spatial distortions (see Chapter 6).

It is desirable to be able to image any anatomical area and therefore patient access is of paramount importance in magnet design.

Magnetic Field Generation

Field generation can be achieved by: permanent magnets or electromagnets. Table 2.1 summarises the advantages and disadvantages of the different magnet types.

Permanent Magnets

Permanent magnets are manufactured from ferromagnetic materials such as iron, nickel or cobalt. They are constructed from blocks of the chosen material and the magnetic field is induced into the blocks at the time of manufacture. Iron is the usual ferromagnetic material used because of its low cost, but it does have the drawback of being very heavy (poor power to weight ratio). One early commercially available 0.3 T magnet weighs 100 tonnes!

No current is required to maintain the magnetic field; the only power requirements are for the other components of the system. Neither is heat produced by the generation of the magnetic field, and so there are no cooling requirements. This results in a system with relatively low running costs.

Temperature variations within the magnet affect the homogeneity of the field and hence image quality, so the temperature of the clinical environment needs to be kept constant.

The magnetic field produced by a permanent magnet is contained within the magnet itself and this type of magnet has a minimal fringe field, which allows these magnets to be sited almost anywhere within a hospital.

Table 2.1. The advantages and disadvantages of different magnet types

Magnet type	Advantages	Disadvantages
Permanent	1. Low capital and running costs 2. No power requirements 3. Small fringe field 4. No liquid gases required for cooling 5. No heat generated 6. Transverse field	1. Limited field strength (about 0.3 T) 2. Very large mass 3. Difficult to shim 4. Only useful for hydrogen imaging
Resistive air core	1. Low capital cost for moderate field 2. Low running costs 3. Coils easily accessible for maintenance 4. Can be switched off 5. No liquid gases for cooling required 6. No vacuum required	1. Moderate field homogeneity (100 p.p.m. over 35 cm) 2. High power requirements (50–70 kW) 3. Water cooling system required. 4. Maximum field strength limited 5. Potential instabilities in magnetic field due to fluctuations in the power supply 6. Only useful for hydrogen imaging 7. Cooling required
Resistive iron core	1. Low capital cost 2. Low running costs 3. Increase in field strength without increasing weight 4. Small fringe fields	1. High power requirements 2. Potential instabilities in magnetic fields
Superconductive	1. High field strengths obtainable 2. High field homogeneity 3. Extremely stable 4. Low power requirements 5. Potential to extend to other isotopes and chemical shift to analyse 6. Adjustable field strength	1. High capital costs 2. High costs for cryogens and their storage 3. Careful handling of cryogens required 4. Coils not easily accessible 5. Problems with the fringe fields

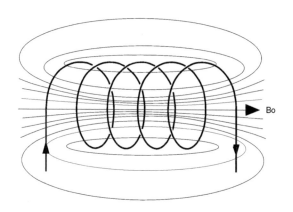

Fig. 2.2. Simple solenoid showing the direction of the generated magnetic field.

Electromagnets

By passing a current through a coil of wire a magnetic field is generated within and around the coil (a simple solenoid: Fig. 2.2).

The electromagnets used in MRI can be divided into two types: resistive magnets and superconducting magnets.

Resistive Magnets. There are two types of resistive magnets: iron core and air core.

The *iron core magnet* is also known as the hybrid system. It consists of a permanent magnet with the addition of conductive windings which enable an increase in magnetic field strength without increasing magnet weight. Copper or aluminium can be used for the windings. Although copper is the better conductor it is heavier and more expensive, so aluminium is preferred.

Iron core magnets are able to produce a relatively high field without the associated problems of large fringe fields. One such system operates at a field strength of 0.4 T.

The *air core magnet* is made by multiple turns of wire (again usually aluminium) wound into a solenoid. The turns of wire are divided into four or six separate coils as shown in Fig. 2.3. The coils have a resistance to the current that passes through them, this generates heat within the system and as a result of this power is lost.

A water cooling system removes excess heat from the magnet but this process has its limitations. As a result there is a limit to the amount of current which can effectively be applied and hence to the maximum field strength which can be achieved in practice.

The fields generated by resistive magnets can be in either the vertical or horizontal direction depending on the orientation of the magnet windings. The field strengths available for air core resistive magnets are 0.01 T up to 0.1 T.

Superconducting Magnets. A superconductor is a material that loses all electrical resistance below a critical temperature. The windings in a superconducting magnet consist of coils of a superconducting alloy of titanium and niobium, embedded in a copper matrix. The copper helps to protect and support the alloy. In the case of a sudden rise in temperature it acts as a heat sink preventing damage to the delicate alloy.

The critical temperature required to produce zero resistance for the alloy is −269 °C (4 K) and this is achieved by immersing the coils in a bath of liquid helium contained in a vessel known as the cryostat. The cryostat thermally insulates the liquid helium. Heat can be transferred to the helium by conduction, convection and radiation. Conduction is minimised by good design and the appropriate choice of materials, while convection is minimised by placing the magnet and surrounding materials in a vacuum. Most of the helium evaporation in a magnet is caused by radiation reaching the magnet windings. This is reduced by surrounding the helium bath with a series of heat shields; the first of these is cooled by the evaporating helium gas, while subsequent shields are cooled by liquid nitrogen or mechanical closed-circuit coolers (refrigeration units).

None of the cryostats is able to prevent evaporation of the liquid helium completely, but they do keep evaporation to a minimum. The helium needs to be topped up periodically to replenish that lost by evaporation. Typically this needs to be carried out every 3–4 months, though the latest generation magnets require only a single helium refill per year. Some manufacturers offer helium reliquefication units which reliquefy the evaporated helium gas and avoid the need for constant topping up. This seems to be the best solution to the problem but it is only recently that such units have proven to be effective.

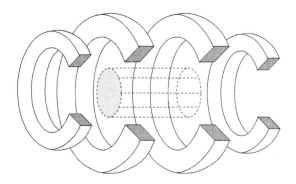

Fig. 2.3. The configuration of an air core magnet.

Magnet Shielding

Because of the very strong magnetic field associated with superconducting magnets there are problems with their siting within the hospital environment. This has three implications: (1) the space required for an independent site, (2) the high cost of building the extra site, and (3) the fringe or stray fields produced in a three-dimensional volume around the magnet and which can have an effect on the surrounding environment.

In the past these problems were overcome by:

1. Building on a green-field site – but this had the obvious inconvenience of being a separate building.
2. Yoke shielding (self shielding), where the magnet is enclosed in a thick iron shield – but this causes an extra burden on the floor as the shield can weigh up to 21 tonnes. However, it will reduce the fringe fields by 50%.
3. Room shielding, where the magnet room is converted into an iron box – but this too is expensive and requires extensive modifications as the shield can be up to 2.5 cm thick and weigh around 50 tonnes.

Recently an alternative method known as active shielding has been developed which reduces the fringe field volume by as much as 95%. Active shielding fea-tures a special array of superconducting coils wound around the outside of the main magnet windings to directly oppose its field. It provides a high degree of shielding with little additional weight. Fig. 2.4 illustrates the reduction in volume of the fringe field compared with a conventional unshielded magnet. This innovation allows for more convenient siting of magnets within the hospital environment, reducing preparatory installation costs dramatically.

Shim Coils

Shimming is the process of eliminating any inhomogeneities within the magnetic field. These inhomogeneities may arise from the magnet or the surroundings in which the magnet is placed.

Shimming is performed using a special probe which can measure magnetic field strength. The probe is placed at multiple predetermined positions within the imaging volume (usually 40–50 cm) and readings taken. Once all the readings (measurements) have been obtained a complex mathematical process called "spherical harmonics expansion" is used to determine the coefficients needed to correct the inhomogeneities.

The correction of these magnetic field inhomo-

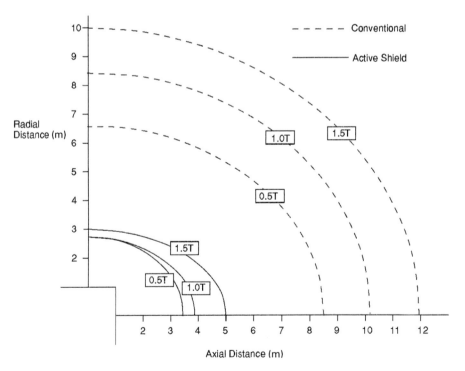

Fig. 2.4. The reduction in the fringe field volume of actively shielded magnet systems.

geneities can be accomplished by either active or passive shimming.

Active Shimming

In active shimming ten to twelve current-carrying shim coils are placed within the bore of the magnet. As each of these receives its own current it generates its own magnetic field. The current required is calculated according to the predetermined coefficients mentioned above and produces an almost perfectly homogeneous field within the bore of the magnet.

In order to prevent interactions (eddy current formation) between shim coils, gradient coils and magnet windings special attention is required in the design of the coils.

Passive Shimming

Passive shimming involves the correction of inhomogeneities by the placement of iron plates inside and/or outside the magnet bore in a standard configuration, the number of plates in each position being determined by a computer program. One manufacturer has recently begun to use iron rods instead of the plates, with a claimed increase in overall homogeneity.

The shimming procedure is carried out during installation and with modern magnets may need checking only if there is evidence of inhomogeneity (i.e. distortion of images). However, if the magnet is used for spectroscopy or any type of research work then it is far more important for the magnetic field to be as homogeneous as possible and shimming should be carried out on a more regular basis. This could mean every day or even, for spectroscopy, before each patient.

Gradient Coils

The gradient coils are situated within the bore of the magnet. A current is passed through the coils, which are designed to produce a linear change in the magnetic field (gradient). Typically the strength of the magnetic field gradients is in the order of 1% of that of the main magnetic field (5–10 millitesla (mT) per metre).

The gradients are positioned in the centre of the main magnet (isocentre). At any point along the axis of the gradient the magnetic field strength is a combination of the main field and the gradient field, as demonstrated in Fig. 2.5. The gradient coils' main role

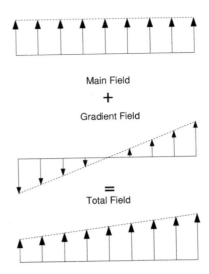

Fig. 2.5. The effect of the gradient magnetic fields on the main magnetic field.

is to encode spatial information onto the MR signal.

It can be seen from the Larmor equation ($\omega_0 = \gamma Bo$) that if a magnetic field gradient is applied along the main field (Bo) the resonance frequencies of the protons will vary according to their position along the gradient (due to the differing field strengths created by the gradient coils). Since the imaging system can measure the frequencies and knows the imposed spatial variations of the main field (created by the gradient coils) the position of the resonating protons can be determined.

The gradient coils produce linear field gradients in all three orthogonal planes (X,Y,Z). If imaging is carried out in a non-orthogonal plane, e.g. coronal oblique, then a combination of two sets of gradient coils is used. There are two main designs of coil used to produce linear field gradients: the Maxwell pair (Helmholtz) and Golay coils.

The Maxwell pair (Fig. 2.6) are composed of two

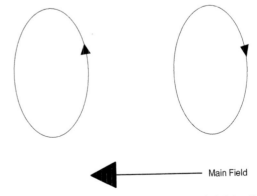

Fig. 2.6. The configuration of Maxwell pair (Helmholtz) coils.

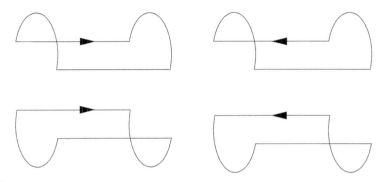

Fig. 2.7. The configuration of Golay coils.

parallel elliptical coils with electrical currents flowing in opposite directions. They are usually positioned at each end of the imaging area and produce gradients along the Z (main field) direction.

The Golay coils (Fig. 2.7) are saddle-shaped coils that consist of two wires with currents flowing in opposite directions. They are used to produce magnetic field gradients along the X and Y directions and can be reversed by simply reversing the current in the coils.

During data acquisition the gradients are switched on and off very rapidly, due to the short imaging times used (milliseconds). It is the switching on and off of the gradients and the rapidly changing magnetic field which cause vibrations of the gradients against the cryostat and make the noise associated with MRI. This rapid switching of the gradients can cause eddy currents to form within the metallic structures of the magnet and cryostat. These eddy currents generate magnetic fields of their own which have a small but significant effect upon the gradients produced and hence upon image quality.

The eddy current effects produce images which are spatially misregistered and often blurred. One way that this is overcome is by the use of self-shielded gradient coils which by design confine their magnetic field to the interior of the coils. Another way of minimising the effect of eddy currents is by a process of precompensating the current which goes to turn on the gradients. This allows the production of a gradient of the correct strength and duration. An eddy current compensation program is used at installation to determine the precise precompensation required.

RF Transmitter/Receiver Coils

As discussed in Chapter 1, resonance is observed in hydrogen nuclei after the application of a magnetic field at 90° to the main magnetic field. This is achieved using a radiofrequency (RF) pulse at the Larmor frequency. The signal produced then needs to be detected to enable image production to take place.

The requirements of the RF coils are: (1) to surround the subject/volume being sampled, (2) to produce a homogeneous RF field across the subject in order to obtain the same flip angle throughout the subject when the coil is energised and (3) to produce a magnetic field at 90° to the main field (Bo).

RF Synthesis

A whole range of radiofrequencies around the Larmor frequency are generated by the RF synthesisers. These frequencies are then amplified by the RF amplifier and transmitted by an RF coil to excite the tissues within the imager.

RF coils can be built as two separate coils: one to transmit the RF pulse and one to receive the MR signal. However, because these processes occur at different times it is possible to use a single coil to both transmit and receive.

The coils are made of wide copper ribbon or tubing, as the RF used in MRI is of such a frequency that it tends to travel on the surface of the conductor used as the coil. The coils are situated in close proximity to the patient within the magnet bore and, when installed in the magnet system, must be tuned to the required frequency of the system.

The RF transmitter coils are usually formed in either a linear or quadrature configuration, depending on the direction of the main magnetic field (i.e. horizontal as in a superconducting magnet or vertical as in most permanent/resistive magnets). Horizontal fields usually employ saddle-shaped (Golay) coils (Fig. 2.8), while vertical fields have solenoid-shaped coils (Fig. 2.9).

Having a quadrature configuration instead of linear configuration improves the efficiency of RF tranmis-

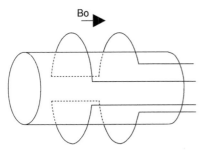

Fig. 2.8. Saddle-shaped (Golay) RF coils.

sion. The quadrature coils consist of two separate coils which operate 90° out of phase from each other and thus generate a rotating field perpendicular to the main magnetic field ($B1$). This is a more efficient way of producing the RF power and can, in theory at least, reduce those requirements by up to 50%. The second benefit of quadrature coils is in the receive mode of the RF system, where they produce an increase in the overall signal detected and have been found to be 40% more efficient than linear receive coils.

Centre Frequency Check

The term centre frequency check refers to the matching of the RF pulse frequency to the frequency of the signal from the tissues being imaged (Larmor frequency). It would be thought that in a homogeneous supercon-ducting magnet system this procedure would be superfluous. However, magnet susceptibility effects of the different tissues can significantly alter the resonance frequency, requiring this check to be undertaken.

A wide range of frequencies are transmitted to the tissues, centred around the theoretical resonant fre-quency, and the receive signal is displayed on the operator's monitor as a graph of frequency versus sig-nal intensity. The operator has the ability to adjust the frequency of the RF pulse so that the signal frequency matches it exactly. On high-field systems two separate peaks are usually visible. These represent the individual

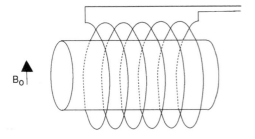

Fig. 2.9. Solenoid-shaped RF coils.

signals detected from fat and water, with the water peak being at the higher frequency. It may be desirable to adjust the RF frequency to either one of these two peaks or mid-way between the two. This procedure is performed at the beginning of every study or when-ever a new area of interest is selected. It contributes greatly to image quality and therefore needs to be per-formed accurately.

Transmitter Adjustment (Tuning)

Transmitter adjustment allows for the calculation of the amount of RF power required to produce the desired flip angles. The adjustment is necessary for every sequence on most systems, although some systems require only one tuning adjustment at the beginning of a study of a specific area.

One of several methods of adjustment is to excite the central slice of the tissue being imaged with RF initially at low power and gradually to increase the RF power in a stepwise manner. The signals are detected until maximum and minimum levels are achieved, representing the 90° and 180° pulses respectively.

If the sequence being undertaken requires flip angles other than 90° or 180° (gradient echo sequence) then the system calculates the amount of power required to produce an intermediate flip angle.

Slice thickness also has a direct effect on the amount of RF power required to produce the correct flip angle. The thicker the slice the more power is required to excite the protons within that slice.

Receive Gain

The signal received is converted by an analogue-to-digital converter (ADC) into a digital form to be analysed by the computer. The ADC can receive sig-nals of only a certain dynamic range, so the receive gain (amplification) must be adjusted so that the signals collected fall within this range. The receive gain is the same as the degree of attenuation of the signal.

The effect of incorrect receive gain setting can be seen in Fig. 2.10.

The Receiver

The signal produced from the resonating protons in MRI is only one billionth of the transmitted RF power. Transverse magnetisation induces an alternat-ing current into the RF receiver coil and the induced signal is then amplified by an RF pre-amplifier. This amplified signal is filtered to produce the difference between the RF transmitted and the signal received.

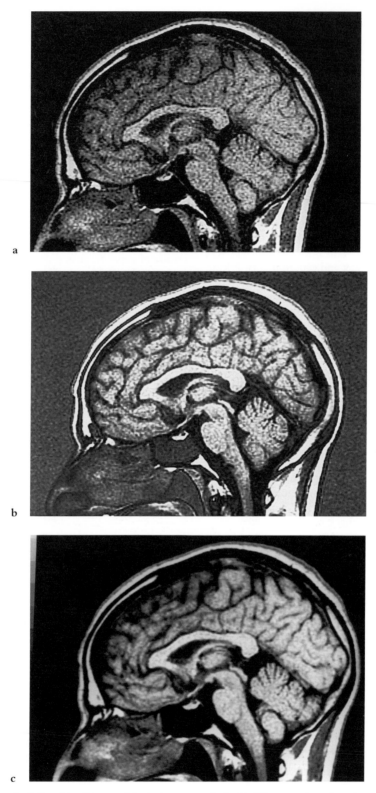

Fig. 2.10a–c   These sagittal T1-weighted images of the brain were acquired with different receive gain settings: **a** too low, **b** too high and **c** correct.

This difference in signal is in the range of audiofrequencies (AF) and it is then amplified by a factor of 10 to 1000 by an AF amplifier. The signal is then directed to an ADC which converts the AF signal into a series of binary numbers that are stored in the computer memory for later manipulation. The RF coil and RF pre-amplifier design predominantly determine the amount of system noise added to the MR signal. It is desirable that this is kept to a minimum as excess noise degrades the information available.

The receiver is tuned to a range of frequencies contained in the MR signal and which is referred to as the "bandwidth". The signal picked up by the receiver coil goes through a bandpass filter to be processed, and this helps to minimise the signals detected from frequencies outside the useful range.

Signal-to-Noise Ratio (SNR)

The signal-to-noise ratio is the ratio between the amount of signal received from the tissue being imaged and the amount of noise generated within the MR system. It is important that the amount of noise is kept to an absolute minimum.

Noise in the MR image is produced by the pickup in the RF coil itself, and improvement in the SNR can be obtained by using specially designed coils in close proximity to the area being imaged, thus picking up a greater signal. These special coils are known as surface coils.

Surface Coils

All areas of the body can be imaged using the head and body RF coils but there are certain times when image quality can be improved dramatically by using surface coils. These are RF coils specially designed to be placed as close as possible to the area of interest (e.g cervical spine, lumbar spine, knee). As well as giving a greater SNR, better-resolution images are possible because there is sufficient signal to use small fields of view in conjunction with large reconstruction matrices.

Surface coils are constructed in a similar way to transmitter coils (copper ribbon or tubing) with the addition of a capacitance circuit in order that the exact matching of the coil to the MR signal can be achieved. As with the transmitter coils they must also produce a secondary magnetic field at 90° to the main field in order to operate efficiently.

It is also important that the coil is "de-coupled" before the RF pulse is emitted, to prevent it from discharging through the coil and causing damage. This de-coupling is achieved automatically by various different methods including crossed diodes.

There are many different surface coil designs available and they are being improved all the time. To some extent their design depends upon the area being imaged; the nearer the coil is to the area under examination the better the signal received. *It is important that the correct selection of coil is made as inappropriate selection could result in insufficient signal being collected, which would produce a noisy non-diagnostic image.*

Fig. 2.11 illustrates the various different designs of coils available. Of particular interest is the recently developed phased array system which enables image acquisition over large fields of view with a better SNR and resolution than the conventional body coil. This

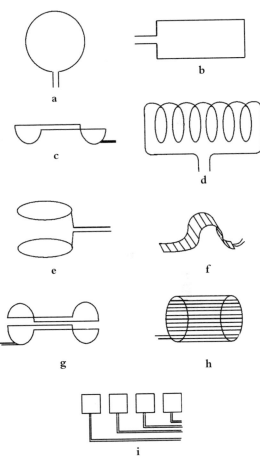

Fig. 2.11a–i The design of various different surface coils. **a** Flat circular coil, used for the temporo-mandibular joint, spine, orbits, musculoskeletal system, etc. **b** Rectangular "licence plate" coil, used mainly for the spine. **c** Half saddle coil, used for neck imaging. **d** Solenoid coil, which must be at 90° to the main magnetic field (Bo) and is mainly used in resistive/permanent magnet systems with vertical fields. **e** Helmholtz pair, used for neck, shoulder and wrists. **f** Flexible linear coil, used for neck and extremities. **g** Saddle coil, used for head and neck imaging at low/mid field strengths. **h** Birdcage quadrature coil, used for head imaging at mid to high field strengths. **i** Phased array coils, used to image the whole spine and pelvis.

Table 2.2. Advantages and disadvantages of different coil types

Coil type	Advantages	Disadvantages	Use
Simple loop	Sensitivity	Depth	Spine, orbits
Saddle shape	Sensitivity; anatomical shape	Depth	Cervical spine
Helmholtz	Homogeneous on small volume	Shape/anatomy	Shoulder
Double saddle	Large volume	Homogeneity	Knee
Standard quadrature	Sensitivity	Homogeneity	Spine
Birdcage quadrature	Sensitivity; homogeneous	Complex	Body/head
Phased array	Sensitivity; large FOV	Complex; extra financial implications due to four times number of receiver parts and extra computer memory to store data collected	Whole spine, pelvis

FOV, field of view.

system comprises several coils arranged as either (1) a linear array, in which a number of coils are positioned end-to-end to enable a long field of view, or (2) a volume array, in which coils are positioned around the area of interest to improve the depth of view. Each coil in the array has its own independent receiver and images are acquired from each coil and reconstructed simultaneously from data stored on separate memory boards. Fig. 2.12 shows the differing sensitivities of various different coil designs.

Table 2.2 shows the advantages and disadvantages of different coil types.

The Computer

The computer system is composed of three main parts: pulse control module, image processor and systems manager.

The Pulse Control Module

The pulse control module controls the precise timing, shape and strength of the RF and gradient pulses in such a way as to produce the recognised MRI pulse sequences. It can also allow manipulation of these pulses for the development of new pulse sequences.

Image Processor

The data received during a pulse sequence are collected and fed into an array processor which reconstructs the data into a two-dimensional image. The images produced are displayed on a cathode ray tube (CRT). The display matrix is most commonly 512×512, with interpolation of data up to this matrix size if a smaller reconstruction matrix has been used (i.e. 256×256).

The image processor has controls to the window and level settings, which are operator defined but according to the signals which have been received by the receiver. The image processor also allows many mathematical functions to be carried out, such as magnification, definition of regions of interest, addition and subtraction.

The images produced are stored on the systems hard (winchester) disc and from there long-term data storage is achieved by magnetic tape or optical laser disc.

Systems Manager

The systems manager manages the various interactions between the subsystems already mentioned, placing their functions/commands in order of priority: i.e. top priority must be given to the pulse sequence controller while a scan is being carried out and the data received must be collected and stored so as not to be missed or lost. In order to achieve this, access to a buffer memory is essential.

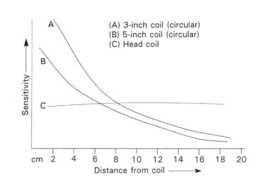

Fig. 2.12. The sensitivities of differently designed surface coils and the way in which sensitivities vary with distance.

3 Pulse Sequences

Pulse sequences have been developed by MR physicists to enable the imaging of the different tissue characteristics presented in MRI. They are precisely timed pulses of radiofrequency (RF) used in conjunction with gradient magnetic fields to produce MR signals.

When considering pulse sequences it is important to become familiar with certain terms which will be used time and again during this chapter. These terms are:

RF Pulse. A brief burst of radiofrequency (at or around the Larmor frequency) delivered to the object being scanned that results in the net magnetisation being rotated away from the direction of the main magnetic field. The strength and duration of the pulse determine the precise rotation of the magnetisation.

TR or Repetition Time. The time between the beginning of one pulse sequence and the beginning of the succeeding pulse sequence.

TE or Echo Time. Time interval from the first RF pulse to the middle of the spin echo or gradient echo production. Essentially this is the time between the RF excitation pulse and the MR signal sampled.

TI or Inversion Time. The time between the initial 180° RF pulse and the 90° RF pulse in an inversion recovery sequence.

Flip Angle. The angle by which the net magnetisation is rotated away from the main magnetic field following an RF pulse.

In the course of the descriptions of the different pulse sequences they will be represented diagrammatically, to aid an understanding of the basic concepts involved.

As previously mentioned pulse sequences have been developed to enable detection of all the different MR parameters and they are being improved all the time. The parameters which can determine contrast are: T1, T2, proton density, T2*, chemical shift, diffusion/perfusion, flow, susceptibility and magnetisation transfer contrast.

When considering the pulse sequences available we shall concentrate mainly on the more commonly used sequences, namely:

Saturation recovery (partial saturation)
Spin echo
Multiple spin echo
Inversion recovery
Gradient echo

We will then briefly consider the more complex sequences available.

Saturation Recovery (Partial Saturation)

Saturation recovery is the simplest pulse sequence and consists of a series of 90° RF pulses with a predetermined equal interval between each pulse, as demonstrated in Fig. 3.1. The 90° pulse rotates the net magnetisation into the transverse plane (relative to the main magnetic field Bo). This transverse magnetisation then decays exponentially to realign itself with the main magnetic field – hence the alternative name for the sequence of repeated free induction decay (FID).

This explanation holds true only if sufficient time is allowed between each RF pulse (TR) to allow complete longitudinal relaxation of the excited tissue. If these criteria are met then the signal following each RF pulse contains information about the tissue's proton density. If the TR is short this results in incomplete longitudinal relaxation before the following RF pulse and therefore the signal is gradually attenuated (partially saturated). It follows, then, that the amplitude of the signal is determined by how much longitudinal relaxation has occurred before the next RF pulse. The resulting signals contain information about T1 of the tissue as well as its proton density.

TR is the only variable in this sequence and it can be altered so that more or less T1 information is contained in the signal. Partial saturation sequences are used predominantly to show anatomical detail.

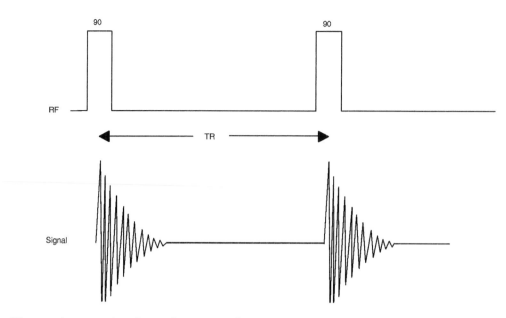

Fig. 3.1. Diagrammatic representation of a saturation recovery pulse sequence showing the RF pulse and the MR signal it produces.

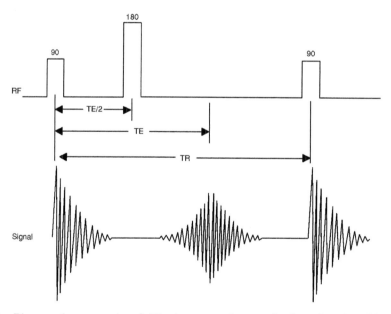

Fig. 3.2. Diagrammatic representation of a SE pulse sequence demonstrating the re-formation of the MR signal (echo).

Spin Echo (SE)

The spin echo sequence uses a 90° RF pulse followed by a second 180° RF pulse as shown in Fig. 3.2, after which the signal is collected. As discussed in Chapter 1, following a 90° RF pulse relaxation occurs both longitudinally and transversely. Immediately following the 90° RF pulse net magnetisation is in the transverse plane, and all the protons contributing to this net magnetisation are in phase (spinning together). However, because of magnetic inhomogeneities, some of these protons will precess at a different rate to others resulting in a gradual loss of phase (loss of phase coherence). The result of this would be a loss of signal.

A second, 180° RF pulse results in a gradual rephas-

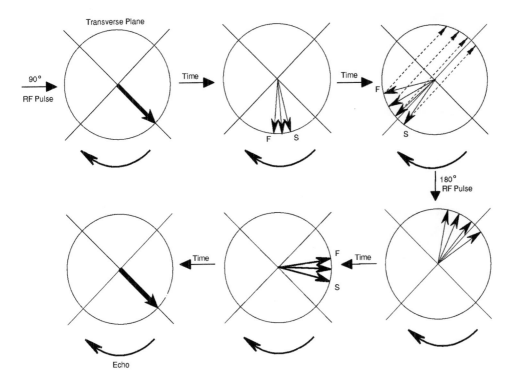

Fig. 3.3. Diagrammatic representation of the loss of phase of the precessing protons in the transverse plane and the effect of the 180° RF pulse in causing rephasing of those protons, forming an echo. F, fast; S, slow.

ing of the protons (proportional to the time after the initial 90° pulse that the 180° pulse is applied). Fig. 3.3 shows the effect of the sequence upon net magnetisation in the transverse plane. The amplitude of the rephased signal will be smaller than the original signal due to the irreversible loss of phase coherence caused by the T2 relaxation process.

The variables in this sequence are TR and TE, and by manipulating these factors it is possible to obtain tissue information that is T1, T2, or proton density weighted. Below are three examples of SE sequences with different TR and TE times.

1. Long TR (2000–4000 ms), short TE (20–30 ms)

Following the 90° RF pulse all the excited protons are allowed to regain their longitudinal net magnetisation completely before the next RF pulse. Even though the excited volume contains different tissues with different T1 times the long TR allows complete longitudinal relaxation of all the tissues.

The tissues in this excited volume will also have different T2 times. If the echo time were longer then the T2 differences would be detected. However, in this case a short TE has been used and so there has been

very little time for any signal decay; therefore differences in neither T1 nor T2 will be detected. Instead the signal detected refers to the amount of hydrogen in the volume. This is known as the "proton density" (Fig. 3.4).

2. Long TR (2000–4000 ms), long TE (80–120 ms)

As in the previous example the long TR allows complete longitudinal relaxation of the excited volume. However, because a longer time elapses before a signal is received (TE) the difference between the T2 relaxation times of different tissues becomes more apparent. The tissues with the longer T2 times make a greater contribution to the overall signal, causing them to appear "bright" on the resulting images.

The correct terminology for these images is "T2-weighted", but they still have some contributing signal from the T1 and proton density of the tissues as shown in Fig. 3.5. T2-weighted sequences are used to demonstrate pathology as diseased tissues have longer T2 times than normal tissues and this sequence highlights these differences.

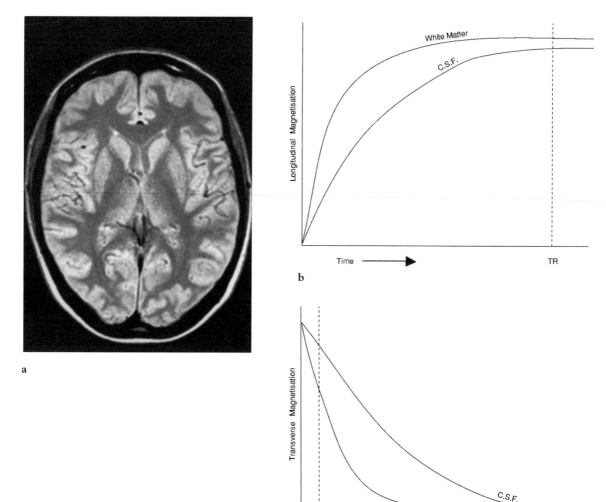

Fig. 3.4 **a** A proton density image of the brain acquired with a long TR (3000 ms) and a short TE (25 ms). The graphs reflect **b** transverse magnetisation and **c** longitudinal magnetisation for the two tissues shown. C.S.F., cerebrospinal fluid.

3. Short TR (450–700 ms), short TE (20–30 ms)

The short TE will not allow enough time for the decay of the transverse magnetisation so variations in T2 will have little effect on the signal intensity. The short TR used means that only those tissues with a short T1 time will have completely recovered their longitudinal magnetisation before the next 90° RF pulse, and so it is these tissues which have the greatest signal to contribute in the transverse plane. They will therefore appear "bright" compared with tissues with a longer T1 which have not completely recovered their longitudinal magnetisation.

The proton density of the tissue still has a part to play in the overall appearance of the image but this

sequence is known as a "T1-weighted" sequence, as demonstrated in Fig. 3.6. T1-weighted images are used predominantly to give anatomical detail about the area under examination.

Multiple Spin Echo

The multiple spin echo sequence is an extension of the spin echo sequence, using further echoes generated by subsequent 180° rephasing pulses as shown in Fig. 3.7. It allows the generation of images all with different tissue contrast. A long TR is usually employed, allowing

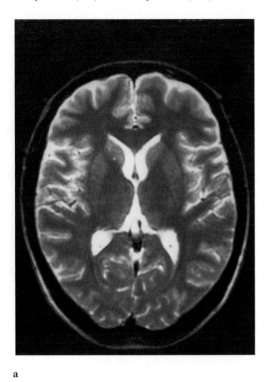

a

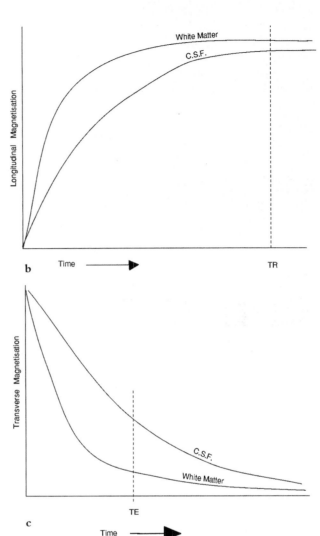

Fig. 3.5 a A SE T2-weighted image of the brain acquired with a long TR (3000 ms) and a long TE (100 ms). **b, c** The graphs indicate the different T2 relaxation characteristics. C.S.F., cerebrospinal fluid.

complete longitudinal relaxation, and TE times are selected according to the information required.

Usually proton density information is obtained from a short TE (say 25 ms) and then subsequent T2-weighted image data after multiples of the first TE (say 50, 75 and 100 ms) are collected. A variation of this sequence is the Variable Echo sequence which allows the collection of two asymmetrical echoes (e.g. 25 and 100 ms). It is obviously a very useful way of obtaining both sets of information (proton density and T2) during the same scanning sequence, because both require long TR times and therefore long scan times.

Fast Spin Echo (FSE) or Turbo Spin Echo (TSE)

The fast or turbo spin echo sequence is one of the latest sequences available and is a modification of the spin echo pulse sequence.

In conventional spin echo imaging the MR signals are stored as raw data prior to image reconstruction, each slice having its own raw data set. The signals for each slice are generated from a predetermined number of rows, according to the number of views in the phase-encoding axis. For each TR, signals are acquired for one row of the raw data, the number of phase-encoding steps (or rows) determining how many times

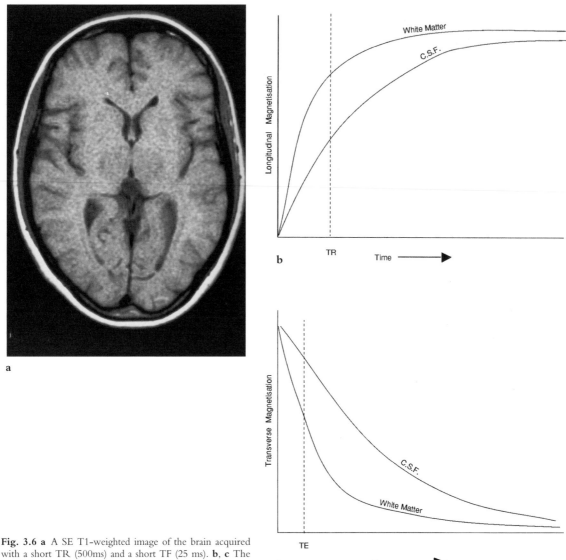

a

Fig. 3.6 a A SE T1-weighted image of the brain acquired with a short TR (500ms) and a short TF (25 ms). **b, c** The graphs show different relaxation characteristics. C.S.F., cerebrospinal fluid.

the TR has to be repeated and thus directly influencing the overall scan time.

The fast spin echo sequence uses a series of 180° RF pulses after the original 90° excitation pulse. This produces a train of echoes (echo train) and for each of the echoes the value of the phase-encoding gradient is changed. Multiple rows of data are acquired during each TR so fewer TRs are required to produce an image, thus reducing the overall scan time.

The length of the echo train is selected by the operator and varies from 2 to 16 echoes. The echo train length (ETL or turbo factor) determines the overall scan time and is a direct measure of the scan time compared with that in a conventional spin echo sequence (e.g. an ETL of 16 would reduce the scan

time by a factor of 16 and an ETL of 4 would reduce the scan time by a factor of 4).

The multiple 180° pulses produce different rows of data that are weighted according to their position along the train, i.e. the first echoes in the train are proton density weighted and the last are heavily T2-weighted, with the intermediate echoes varying accordingly. The way that the contrast in the images is controlled is related to the values of the phase-encoding gradients given to the different echoes in the train. High phase-encoding gradient values provide the detail and low phase-encoding gradient values provide the intensity pattern in the final image. By controlling the phase-encoding gradient values it is therefore possible to decide whereabouts in the train the intensity

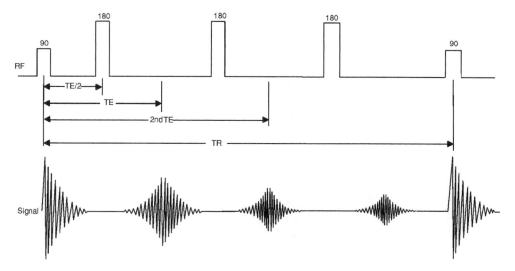

Fig. 3.7. Multiple SE pulse sequence.

pattern of the image is centred and where the detail of the image is obtained.

An effective TE is selected by the operator and the sequence centres the low phase-encoding gradient values to the echoes around that TE. This results in the echoes collected around that TE having most influence on the signal intensity and therefore determining contrast in the final image. The echoes furthest away from the selected TE are given the largest phase-encoding values and contribute least to the signal the intensities of the image but most to the detail within the image.

The contrast produced on fast spin echo images is similar to that produced in conventional spin echo images (compare Fig. 3.8a,b). There are some subtle differences but these go beyond the scope of this text.

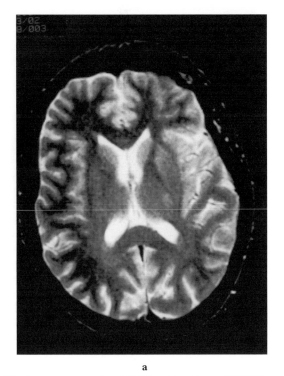

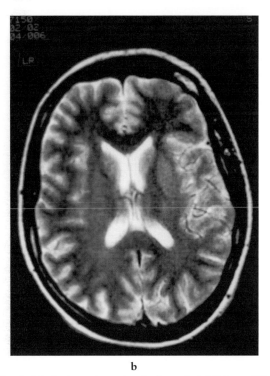

a

b

Fig. 3.8. a A conventional SE T2-weighted image (TR 2000 ms, TE 85 ms) of the brain, total scan time 9 minutes. **b** A FSE image (TR 2000 ms, effective TE 85 ms, ETL 16) of the brain, total scan time 34 seconds!

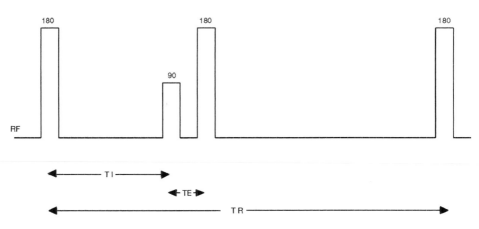

Fig. 3.9. An IR pulse sequence.

The important advantage of the fast spin echo sequence is that it opens the possibility of additional sequences being performed in an acceptable examination time (e.g. fast spin echo T2-weighted sequences in additional planes, a three-dimensional volume acquisition or an MR angiography sequence). Another option which becomes practicable using the fast spin echo sequence is the use of a 512 reconstruction matrix, which gives greatly improved in-plane resolution.

Inversion Recovery (IR)

The inversion recovery sequence uses a 180° RF pulse to invert the net magnetisation so as to directly oppose the main magnetic field. The net magnetisation then recovers its longitudinal magnetisation. After a certain prescribed time (TI) a 90° RF pulse is applied followed by a second 180° RF pulse (to rephase the transverse magnetisation) and an echo is received (TE), as demonstrated in Fig. 3.9.

Methods of Reconstruction

There are two types of image reconstruction used with the inversion recovery sequence.

In phase-corrected or real reconstruction the initial 180° RF pulse in the inversion recovery sequence inverts the net magnetisation and over time, as previously described, the different tissues realign at different rates with the main magnetic field. The phase-corrected images can detect whether the longitudinal component of the tissues is positive or negative (Fig. 3.10)

and assign a pixel value accordingly. This produces images with a large dynamic range.

Magnitude reconstruction, in contrast, is able to detect only the strength (magnitude) of the signal and cannot differentiate between the signal's negative or positive values. The dynamic range is only half that of phase-corrected reconstruction.

Timing Factors

The inversion recovery sequence has three variable timing factors that can be manipulated to achieve the desired results: TR, TI and TE.

Changing TR

Usually a TR of three times the T1 of the tissues being imaged is selected to allow complete recovery of the longitudinal magnetisation. The TR times generally used with an inversion recovery sequence do not usually allow complete recovery of those substances with a long T1 (e.g. cerebrospinal fluid and urine), but this can be used to advantage by giving better contrast between the long T1 fluids and their immediate surroundings (e.g. brain in the case of cerebrospinal fluid).

Using a TR of less than three times the T1 of the tissues being imaged means that those tissues with a longer T1 will have insufficient time to relax completely before the next excitation pulse and thus have less signal to contribute to the overall image. A short TR can therefore be used to reduce the relative signal intensity of tissues with a long T1 such as spleen.

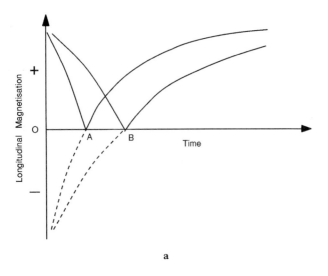

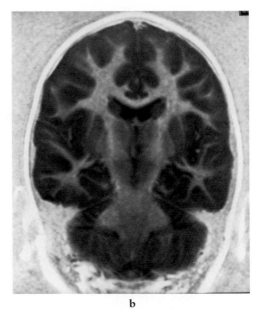

Fig. 3.10 a The longitudinal magnetisation over time showing the relaxation of two different tissues in an IR sequence. The phase corrected image (*dashed line*) can differentiate between the sign of magnetisation which generates improved tissue contrast. **b** Phase-corrected reconstruction of a coronal brain scan (TR 2000 ms, TI 400 ms, TE 30 ms) showing superb grey/white matter differentiation.

Changing TI

TI can be either short (0–250 ms), medium (250–700 ms) or long (700 ms or more).

Short TI. The short TI IR (STIR) sequence can be used in many instances as an alternative to standard spin echo sequences producing high net tissue contrast. Following the 90° pulse the T1 and T2 contrast are additive which enhances the contrast between the different tissues. Since pathological tissue has a characteristic increase in both T1 and T2 the short TI IR sequence can be used to highlight these tissues very effectively.

By carefully selecting the TI so that the signal intensity of a particular tissue is zero at the time of the 90° RF pulse (typically 56%–69% of a tissue's T1 if TR is greater than three times the tissue's T1), then the signal from that tissue is "suppressed" and contributes nothing to the resultant image. A TI of between 80 and 150 ms achieves fat suppression and this can be useful when imaging the orbit, abdomen and various soft tissue lesions. This is demonstrated in Fig. 3.11, which compares a conventional spin echo image with a STIR image. The same principle can be used to suppress the signal from other tissues (i.e. white matter at approximately 250 ms) but its use is predominantly as a technique for fat suppression.

Suppression of subcutaneous abdominal fat is very useful for minimising the effects of respiratory artifact, as it is the high signal from fat which emphasises this artifact.

Medium TI. Medium TI inversion recovery sequences are used to give excellent T1 contrast between different tissues. It is recommended that TI times are midway between the T1 values of the two tissues that need to be differentiated.

This sequence is most often used in the imaging of the brain as it gives good contrast between the grey and white matter. It is used in conjunction with phase-corrected reconstruction to bring out the contrast between the two tissues even further, as shown in Fig. 3.10. The TE for this sequence is kept to a minimum (25–30 ms) to maintain its T1 dependence.

Long TI. As there is a general increase in the T1 values of tumours and the surrounding oedema this sequence is useful in differentiating between the two. It can also be used in paediatric brains due to the normal three- or fourfold increase in T1 relative to the adult brain.

In the same way that a short TI can be selected to suppress the signal from fat, a recent application of a long TI sequence suppresses the signal from cerebrospinal fluid (CSF) and other fluids. Typical TI values of 1800–3000 ms are used and a TR of 6000 ms will allow complete longitudinal relaxation of all tissues. The TE selected will vary according to the information required. A short TE would yield a proton density weighted image and a long TE would give a T2-weighted image. CSF, because of its long T2 and high signal on T2-weighted images, can sometimes mask lesions in the immediate vicinity of CSF collections, i.e. periventricular lesions in the white matter.

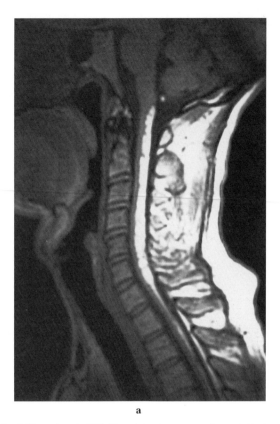
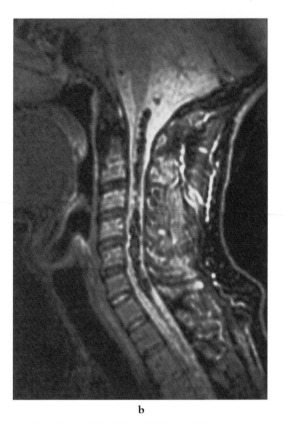

a   b

Fig. 3.11 **a** A sagittal SE T1-weighted sequence of a cervical spine demonstrating a lipoma (TR 500 ms, TE 21 ms). **b** Same patient using a STIR sequence which shows its effect by suppressing the fat (TR 2000 ms, TI 100 ms, TE 25 ms).

This sequence can be used to differentiate such lesions as well as giving greater lesion conspicuity in other ways.

Because CSF is a flowing substance nulling the signal from it can also be useful when imaging the spine, and this sequence has been shown to be equally useful in demonstrating spinal pathology. The acronym for the sequence is FLAIR, which stands for FLuid Attenuated Inversion Recovery sequence. Fig. 3.12 shows an example of the sequence.

Changing TE

As with SE sequences, increasing TE increases the T2 weighting of the image.

For short TI sequences a longer TE can be used in order to image tissues with a longer T2 (i.e. kidneys and brain). STIR sequences utilise the T1-dependent contrast of the tissues and so require a shorter TE. When using medium TI the TE should be kept to a minimum to maintain the sequence's T1 dependence. For long TI sequences the TE can be increased to affect the relative T2 weighting of the images.

Fast Inversion Recovery

A fast inversion recovery sequence has recently been introduced which uses the fast spin echo sequence following the 180° inversion pulse. This reduces acquisition times considerably and so makes the sequence more practicable. It can be used with a short, medium or long TI and its full potential is still being evaluated.

Gradient Echo

Gradient echo techniques incorporate a whole family of different pulse sequences which rely on a reduced flip angle and a short TR to enhance different image contrasts. They have been developed to provide rapid acquisition – in the order of seconds rather than the minutes required for the more conventional acquisition methods. There are numerous reasons to want to acquire data quickly: to minimise patient discomfort, to minimise movement/respiration artifacts and to improve throughput. There is also the possible appli-

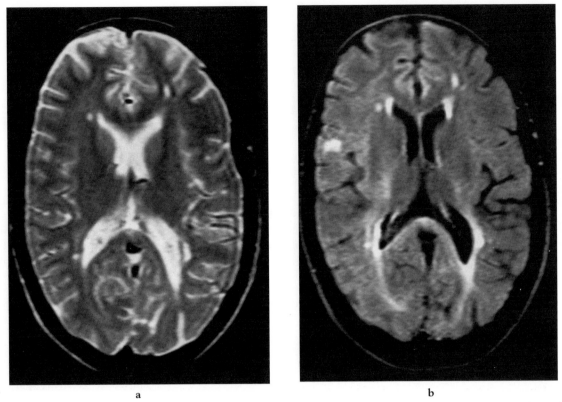

Fig. 3.12   **a** An axial SE T2-weighted sequence of the brain demonstrating multiple white matter lesions (TR 2503 ms, TE 80 ms). **b** An axial FLAIR sequence in the same patient gives improved conspicuity of the lesions, particularly those in the periventricular region (TR 6511 ms, TI 1800 ms, TE 160 ms). (Courtesy of Picker International Ltd.)

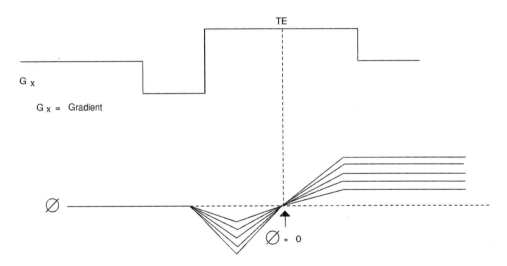

Fig. 3.13.   The mechanism of gradient echo formation. The gradient reversal rephases all the spins giving maximum signal at echo time TE.

cation of the sequence to allow dynamic studies of organs.

With conventional spin echo imaging a 90° pulse is used followed by a 180° rephasing pulse to form the echo. The gradient echo pulse sequence uses flip angles of less than 90°. The 180° rephasing pulse is no longer used and is replaced by reversal of the magnetic field gradient which refocuses the signal in the transverse plane, hence the name "gradient echo". This is shown in Fig. 3.13. More than one RF pulse is of course used in a gradient echo pulse sequence. This has the result of a stimulated spin echo formation which combines with the FID produced by each RF pulse to form the echo.

It can be seen from Fig. 3.13 that rephasing is complete when the time duration of the second gradient pulse is equal to the time duration of the first gradient pulse. Fig. 3.14 shows an example of a gradient echo pulse sequence with the appropriate gradient timings. It is important to understand that the use of a flip angle of less then 90° means that both longitudinal and transverse magnetisation is present.

Table 3.1. Types of gradient echo sequences

Gradient echo sequence	Acronyms	Contrast possible
Steady state	GRASS, FISP, T2 FFE	T2*/T1
Spoiled	SPGR, FLASH, T1 FFE	T1, proton density
Contrast-enhanced	CE-FAST, PSIF	T2

Types of Gradient Echo Sequences

Gradient echo sequences are referred to in various different ways by various different machine manufacturers according to the particular design of pulse sequence used. Basically the sequences can be divided into three categories: (1) steady state gradient echoes, (2) spoiled gradient echoes and (3) contrast-enhanced gradient echoes. Table 3.1 shows the different acronyms by which these sequences are known and the contrast they produce.

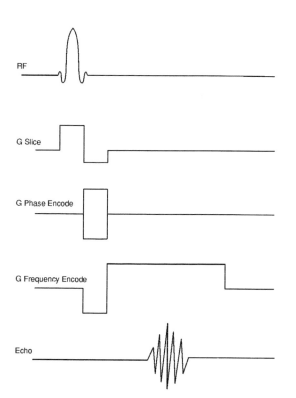

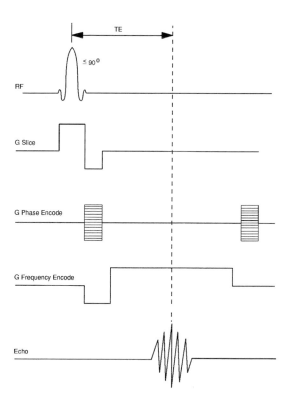

Fig. 3.14. A gradient echo pulse sequence. This diagram differs from the previous pulse sequence diagram in that it also includes the gradient switching.

Fig. 3.15. A gradient echo pulse sequence including the application of the second rewinding phase-encoding gradient pulse.

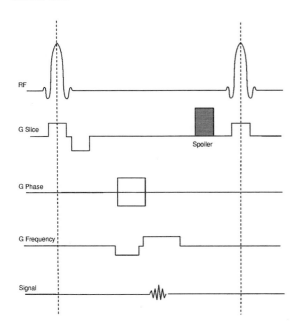

Fig. 3.16. Application of the spoiler gradient during the gradient echo pulse sequence.

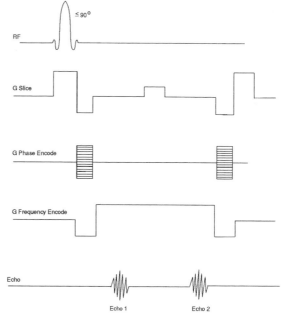

Fig. 3.17. A contrast-enhanced gradient echo sequence.

Steady State Gradient Echo (GRASS, FISP, T2 FFE)

The term steady state refers to the condition which occurs when longitudinal and transverse magnetisation coexist. A "rewinder" gradient pulse is used with this sequence as shown in the pulse sequence diagram in Fig. 3.15. This rewinder pulse is applied on the phase-encoding gradient on those tissues which retain transverse magnetisation. This refocuses their magnetisation, reducing phase artifacts and producing images of higher signal-to-noise ratio (SNR) and greater contrast.

Spoiled Gradient Echo (FLASH, SPGR, T1 FFE)

Spoiled gradient echo sequences differ from the steady state sequences in that a gradient is applied after data acquisition to spoil or destroy any residual transverse magnetisation. Fig. 3.16 demonstrates where the spoiler gradient is applied during the gradient echo pulse sequence. Since this sequence uses spoiler gradients to destroy the residual transverse magnetisation T2 dependence is almost entirely eliminated. Alternatively, the spoiling can be achieved with RF pulses, although this has the disadvantage of increasing the specific absorption rate (SAR; see Chapter 9). The result of spoiling is that the sequence produces images which are either proton density weighted or T1-weighted or a combination of both.

Contrast-Enhanced Gradient Echo (CE-FAST, PSIF, SSFP, T2 FFE)

The normal steady state gradient echo sequence produces contrast with a mixture of T2 and T1. A further pulse sequence developed allows the MR signal to produce much stronger T2 contrast. With contrast-enhanced gradient echo sequences two echoes are produced. The first, reflecting longitudinal magnetisation, is produced immediately following the RF pulse, while the second, which reflects the transverse magnetisation, is collected immediately before the next RF excitation. It is this second echo collected which is T2 weighted. Fig. 3.17 shows the pulse sequence diagram for this sequence.

Contrast in Gradient Echo Sequences

Contrast in gradient echo sequences is much more complicated than the contrast generated by spin echo pulse sequences. A third operator-definable parameter, the flip angle, is available and plays a major role in image contrast for this sequence.

Steady State Gradient Echo

If TR is shorter than T2 then the steady state will exist and would favour those tissues with a long T2 (liquids such as CSF, urine and blood), resulting in them appearing bright on the images. Tissues with a shorter T2 (muscle, brain, etc.) would appear dark in comparison. Fat, however, has a long T2/T1 ratio and so appears relatively bright (but not as bright as liquids). For stationary fluids maximum contrast is acquired using large flip angles, but flow disrupts the steady state and therefore for moving fluids such as CSF smaller flip angles (5°–25°) are more appropriate.

For TR times much longer than T2 the sequence changes in its contrast characteristics and becomes almost identical to the spoiled gradient echo sequence.

If long TE times are used with this sequence the images become T2* weighted. Gradient echo sequences do not refocus dephasing caused by inhomogeneities in the main magnetic field (unlike the spin echo's 180° rephasing pulse) and so the dephasing of transverse magnetisation is a function of T2* rather than T2. Long TE times, however, produce artifacts from inhomogeneities and motion.

Spoiled Gradient Echo

When small flip angles are used, even with short TR times, complete longitudinal relaxation will be achieved between each RF pulse. As a result the T1 of different tissues cannot be differentiated and so images would be proton density weighted.

As flip angles increase so the T1 relaxation times of the tissues become more influential on image contrast, with the images becoming more and more T1 weighted.

If TE is increased the images become influenced by the T2* of the tissues.

Contrast-Enhanced Gradient Echo

Only the second echo of the contrast-enhanced sequence is used and it produces strongly T2-weighted images. The TE for this sequence is actually longer than TR (equal to $2 \times TR - TE$). This occurs because the signal from one RF excitation is refocused during a subsequent excitation.

The signals produced from this sequence may be unacceptably low because there may be only a small portion of transverse magnetisation present. The sequence is much less prone to magnetic susceptibility artifacts.

Rapid Gradient Echo (Turbo Flash, Fast SPGR, Turbo FFE, MP-RAGE)

Recent advances in MR equipment have allowed even more rapid switching of the gradients, which makes it possible to obtain images using very short TR times in the order of 4–8 ms and TE times of 2–4 ms. This allows the acquisition of high-resolution images in less than 1 second. The images acquired at such short TR times are predominantly proton density weighted. It is possible, by reducing the number of phase-encoding steps, to acquire images in as little as 150 ms, but unfortunately the resolution of these images is degraded.

A modification of this technique is the use of preparatory RF pulses which alter the longitudinal magnetisation as desired before the sequence itself begins. This allows the operator to choose the desired contrast required. Examples of the usual preparatory pulses used are a 180° inversion pulse producing T1 weighting or a 90°/180°/90° combination which is used to produce T2 contrast.

Three-Dimensional Gradient Echo Imaging

Three-dimensional (3D) imaging is a method of producing multiple thin contiguous slices in a volume of tissue. Normal two-dimensional (2D) imaging does not allow contiguous slices and, because of the strain which would be placed on the gradients, slices of less than 3 mm cannot be achieved. The 3D imaging sequence approaches this problem by exciting the whole volume of tissue with each RF pulse and performing phase encoding in two axes (the normal phase-encoding axis and the slice select axis). Slice thickness can be as small as 1 mm.

The fact that phase encoding in the 3D sequence takes place in two planes means that the overall scan time is increased, as shown in the equations below:

> For a 2D sequence:
> Total scan time = TR × NSA × NPE
>
> For 3D sequence:
> Total scan time = TR × NSA × NPE × NSL

where TR is the repetition time, NPE the number of phase-encoding steps, NSL the number of slices within the volume and NSA the number of signal averages (NEX).

In 3D spin echo imaging the longer TR times used would mean that to obtain the required number of slices only low-resolution images could be produced with scan times of approximately 30 minutes. The gradient echo sequences described previously allow the use of very short TR times and so used in a 3D

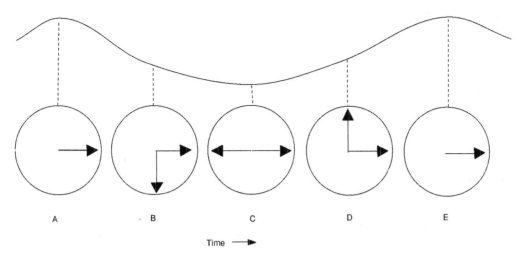

Fig. 3.18. Representation of initially constructive (in-phase) and later destructive (out-of-phase) signal addition as seen in two different spectral components resonating at different frequencies.

sequence the scan times can be dramatically reduced, with high-resolution images possible in scan times of 5–12 minutes.

Features of Gradient Echo Scans

Chemical Shift Effect

In the normal course of events the gradient reversal would be expected to achieve rephasing of all the precessing protons (in the selected slice). However, the protons in water and lipids have slightly different resonant frequencies (3.5 p.p.m.) and so exact rephasing cannot occur. This is referred to as "chemical shift" and it can be used to some advantage in certain circumstances.

Immediately after the RF pulse all the protons are in phase. They then begin to precess at slightly different rates, as described above, and this results in the gradual loss of phase of the two components, as represented in Fig. 3.18. The signals from the two components in phase are summed and 180° out of phase they subtract, so in tissues where there are equal quantities of fat and water the net signal is cancelled. It is therefore the echo time for a particular field strength which determines the relative phases of the two components and to achieve cancellation the following formula can be applied:

$$\text{TE to achieve cancellation of signal} = 3.3/Bo$$

Where Bo is measured in tesla. This gives the following TE times for different field strengths: 11 ms at 0.3 T, 7 ms at 0.5 T, 3.3 ms at 1.0 T and 2.2 ms at 1.5 T.

For both components to be in phase these TE times need to be doubled.

T2* components also affect the signal, but these effects become less significant when short TE times are used (if field strength allows it).

The chemical shift phenomenon was first described when used in conjunction with the partial saturation sequence and its theory of operation has merely been applied to the gradient echo sequence.

Fig. 3.19 shows both in-phase and out-of-phase images of a lumbar spine in a patient with metastases.

Susceptibility

Magnetic susceptibility can be defined as the extent to which materials are magnetised when exposed to a magnetic field. Tissues, depending upon their composition, can vary in their susceptibility and change the effective field for the surrounding protons. The magnetic properties of tissues are characterised by their susceptibility. There are three types of susceptibility: diamagnetic, paramagnetic and ferromagnetic.

Diamagnetic. A diamagnetic substance (e.g. air, water) causes a slight *decrease* in the magnetic field it is placed in (negative susceptibility). Water has a magnetic susceptibility of approximately 13 p.p.m., compared with the other constituents of most tissues which have a magnetic susceptibility of 1 p.p.m. Therefore, depending upon their exact composition, tissues can have varying susceptibilities.

The largest difference in diamagnetic susceptibility occurs between water and air. The difference is

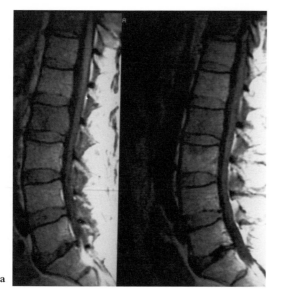 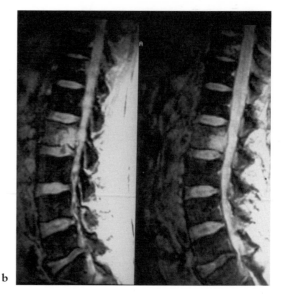

Fig. 3.19 a A sagittal SE T1-weighted image of the lumbar spine in a patient with suspected metastases (TR 500 ms, TE 21 ms). The vertebral body of L2 appears slightly expanded and is of a slightly lower signal intensity than the rest of the vertebra. **b** The same patient using the phase difference gradient echo sequence (TR 580 ms, TE 21 ms, flip 90° [at 0.5 T]). As can be seen there is high signal in the L3 vertebral body due to a change in the proportion of fat and water present, representing a metastatic deposit.

significant enough to cause the protons within the environment of a fluid/air interface to dephase rapidly and, because there is no 180° pulse in the gradient echo sequence, this causes signal loss. This is particularly significant in the nasopharynx, mastoid air cells and other sinuses, and also in other air-filled cavities such as the chest and bowel.

The choice of echo times to some degree determines the amount of artifact present. A long TE would result in a greater amount of susceptibility artifact than a shorter TE.

Paramagnetic. A paramagnetic substance causes a slight *increase* in the magnetic field it is placed in (positive magnetic susceptibility). For example, the breakdown products of haematomas (deoxyhaemoglobin, methaemoglobin and haemosiderin) all give rise to characteristic susceptibility effects on images.

This effect can be used to advantage because gradient echo scans are very sensitive to magnetic susceptibility effects and therefore detection of calcification and small quantities of haemosiderin is possible. Fig. 3.20 demonstrates this feature.

Ferromagnetic. A ferromagnetic substance causes a large *increase* in the magnetic field it is placed in (positive susceptibility). This would be encountered in hip prostheses, surgical clips, dentures, etc., and cause dramatic distortion artifacts.

Echo Planar Imaging (EPI)

Echo planar imaging is, to date, the quickest way of producing an MR image, allowing scan times as low as 30 ms! The acquisition is obtained by a single RF excitation. A train of gradient echoes is generated by using an oscillating gradient technique in which multiple reversals of the frequency-encoding gradient take place. Each of these echoes produced needs to be phase encoded and usually 64–128 phase-encoding steps are employed, leading to scan times of 30–100 ms.

This method puts great demand upon the gradient and transceiver system (very rapid gradient switching and signal sampling) and therefore requires specialised hardware which is not available for use with commercial MR systems at present. However, this hardware is being developed and no doubt will soon become available commercially.

The fact that EPI produces images so quickly means that "snapshot" images of rapidly moving organs (e.g. cine cardiac studies) and perfusion studies are possible.

Magnetisation Transfer Contrast Imaging (MTC)

Magnetisation transfer contrast imaging is also known as dynamic nuclear polarisation.

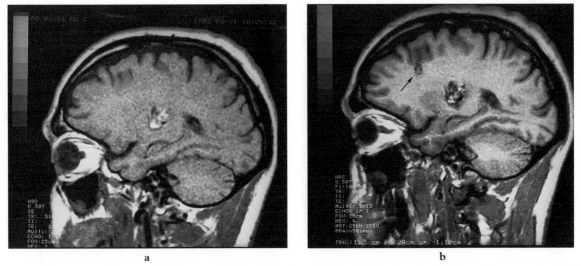

Fig. 3.20.a   A sagittal SE T1-weighted image of the brain (TR 510 ms, TE 21 ms). There is only one obvious lesion present on the SE image. **b** The same patient using a gradient echo sequence (TR 400 ms, TE 12 ms, flip 100°). A second lesion is now visible (*arrow*) due to the increased sensitivity of the sequence to the paramagnetic effect of haemosiderin present in the rim of the lesion.

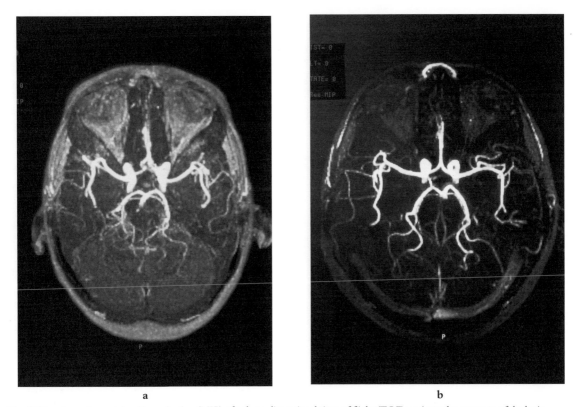

Fig. 3.21.a A maximum intensity projection (MIP) of a three-dimensional time of flight (TOF) angiography sequence of the brain.
b A MIP of a three-dimensional time of flight TOF angiography sequence of the brain used in conjunction with magnetisation transfer contrast. Note the improved background suppression allowing better visualisation of the more peripheral vessels.
(Courtesy of Picker International Ltd.)

There are two types of hydrogen present in the body: (1) free hydrogen (Hf), such as is found in water or CSF, and (2) rigid hydrogen (Hr), which is bound in macromolecules of proteins and membranes (e.g. muscle, cartilage). So far we have discussed only the effect of the RF pulse on Hf. However, there is an interaction between the magnetisation from the Hf in the water and the Hr in the tissues; this effect is known as magnetisation transfer (MT). The magnetisation is transferred by cross-relaxation and chemical exchange.

MT occurs when applying an off-resonance RF pulse to the slice before the conventional 90° pulse of the sequence, thereby saturating the Hr which has a wider range of resonance frequencies. The Hr stores some of this energy and then later (within seconds) transfers it to the Hf. This transfer of energy results in saturation of those Hf protons which in turn lowers the signal from that tissue.

The contrast generated by MT is governed by the proportion of Hf and Hr within the individual tissues. CSF, fluids and lesions with a high water content will experience little signal change because they contain little Hr. Those tissues which contain a high proportion of both Hr and Hf (e.g. muscle, cartilage, grey matter, white matter) will experience the greatest signal loss due to MT.

Applications

This technique can already be used in many situations and is being further evaluated. It will give excellent contrast between cartilage and synovial fluid and is therefore showing some promise for imaging joints. It is proving useful in the evaluation of white matter diseases and showing some promise in both cardiac and abdominal imaging. Magnetic resonance angiography (MRA) can also benefit from the technique as the signal from the background tissue is lowered in time of flight techniques and the vessels stand out against the background. There is also an increase in the conspicuity of the smaller vessels (Fig. 3.21).

4 Image Production

In MRI the signal is derived from resonating hydrogen nuclei: the greater the number resonating, the greater the signal. The signal produced is detected by the receiver or body/head coil and analysed by the computer in order to locate spatially the data acquired.

Images produced in MRI represent slices in various preselected planes through the patient's body. Each slice of tissue is composed of a number of volume elements or voxels. It is displayed in a two-dimensional form on a monitor. The voxels are represented by picture elements or pixels.

As described in Chapter 1 the resonant frequency of the precessing hydrogen protons (Larmor frequency) is determined by the field strength. It therefore follows that if a magnetic field gradient (the gradient fields are produced by the gradient coils, as described in Chapter 2) is applied which alters the field strength across the excited slice, then the protons will resonate at a frequency according to their position along the applied gradient. The signal detected will contain a range of frequencies and amplitudes, frequencies corresponding to the range of field strengths, amplitude to the number of protons contributing to the signal.

The commonest method of analysing this very complex signal is by a mathematical process known as a Fourier transformation (FT) which we will discuss later in this chapter. Early imaging techniques, now no longer used, detected signals from either an individual voxel (single point method), a line of voxels (line method) or a single plane of voxels (planar method). Another method of signal analysis is projection reconstruction. This closely resembles CT reconstruction and uses the well-established algorithm from CT in the reconstruction process, in which a rotating gradient produces multiple projections or views at different angles of rotation. However, this process is very sensitive to motion artifacts and field inhomogeneities and so is not used by modern imaging systems.

Spatial Location of the MR Image

The three pairs of gradient coils built into the MR system (as described in Chapter 2) are used to locate the signal spatially in order to form the familiar MR images. Each of these pairs of coils is used to determine the position and thickness of the excited slice and also to localise the signals produced from that slice. The three coils are labelled according to the axis in which they produce a magnetic field and are given X, Y and Z coordinates:

The Z *coils* (slice select) create a magnetic field gradient along the *length of the magnet bore*.

The Y *coils* (phase-encoding) create a magnetic field gradient from *left to right*.

The X *coils* (frequency-encoding or readout) create a magnetic field gradient *superior to inferior*.

When considering their function we will be acquiring a set of axial images and describing the action of the gradients. Obviously if another plane were to be imaged then the function of each of the gradients would change accordingly.

Slice Selection Excitation

To enable the production of slice images within a volume of tissue a method is needed that restricts the RF excitation to only that pre-selected slice of tissue. This is achieved by the use of a gradient magnetic field perpendicular to the plane of the slice. This means that according to the Larmor equation the resonant frequency of protons will vary depending on their position along the axis of the imposed gradient.

If RF energy of a specific frequency (or a narrow range of frequencies) is applied to the tissue volume, only the protons in the tissue corresponding to the frequency of the RF pulse as determined by the magnetic field gradient will be excited.

The thickness of the slice is directly related to the RF bandwidth and the amplitude of the gradient, as shown in the equation below:

$$F = H \times G \times \text{Slice thickness}$$

where F is the frequency of the RF pulse (Hz), H is the Larmor frequency of hydrogen (Hz/Gauss), G is the gradient amplitude (Gauss/cm) and slice thickness is in centimetres.

Slice Position

The zero point of the gradient coils is the isocentre of the magnet. With this in mind it is possible to excite a slice which is not at the isocentre by changing one of two things: (1) the zero point of the slice selection gradient or (2) the frequency of the RF pulse so that it corresponds to a resonant frequency which is either higher or lower than the resonant frequency at the isocentre of the magnet. The latter method is employed owing to the technical difficulties in rapidly changing the zero position along the slice selection gradient axis.

Slice Profile

Ideally the shape of the slice profile should be rectangular. This would ensure the same amount of RF power is induced across the whole of the excited slice resulting in the same flip angle being produced across the slice too. To ensure that the slice profile is rectangular a mathematical function called a sinc (sin $(x)/x$) is used to modulate the waveform of the RF pulse. The Fourier transform of this function is a rectangle, as shown in Fig. 4.1.

For this rectangular shape to be achieved, however, the sinc pulse must be of infinite duration and this is not possible in practice. Shorter RF pulses produce imperfect slice profiles which results in variation of flip angle across the slice. It may also result in "cross-talk" between the slices if narrow interslice intervals (gaps) are used. Each slice is contaminated with RF from the

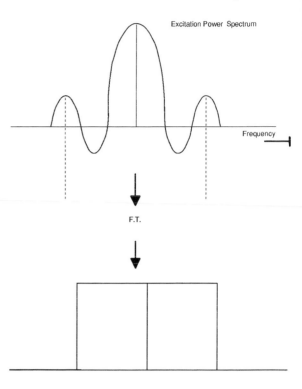

Fig. 4.1. The Fourier transform (FT) of the slice profile.

edges of the adjoining slice profiles. This means that the effective TR for each slice is less than the TR selected for the pulse sequence by the operator.

Cross-talk becomes most apparent in T2-weighted images when tissues with a long T1 (e.g. cerebrospinal fluid) will give a reduced signal as insufficient time is allowed for complete longitudinal relaxation between excitations. An interslice gap of at least 50% of the slice thickness will eliminate this problem (Fig. 4.2). However, as T1-weighted images are less susceptible to cross-talk an interslice gap of 20%–30% of slice thickness is sufficient in this case.

Once excited, the signals from within the slice would be picked up as one composite signal. A way therefore needs to be found of breaking up this composite signal and determining from which point in the slice the signal has come. To achieve this spatial location within the excited slice the Y and X magnetic field gradients are activated independently. These gradients produce: (1) a change in the phase of precession of the excited protons and (2) a change in the frequency of precession of the excited protons. They are therefore labelled the phase-encoding gradient (Y) and the frequency-encoding gradient or readout gradient (X).

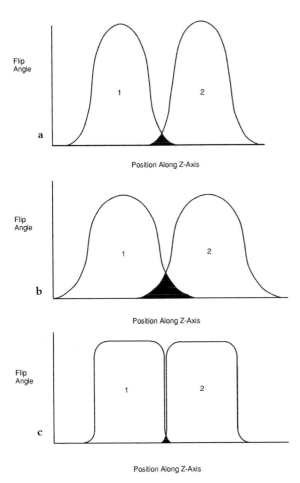

Fig. 4.2a–c. Three slice profiles. **a** is produced by a sinc pulse of moderate duration, **b** by a sinc pulse of shorter duration. Cross-talk between slices 1 and 2 is apparent in both cases but is greater in **b** owing to its poorer slice profile. Cross-talk can be reduced by increasing the interslice gap. Long sinc pulses or computer-optimised RF pulses produce nearly rectangular slice profiles (**c**), permitting much smaller interslice gaps. (Courtesy of R.R. Edelman and J.R. Hesselink.)

Once this process has taken place it is repeated a number of times, each time with an identical change in the amplitude of the magnetic field gradient. For every step in amplitude a different set of signals is obtained, differing only in respect of their phase.

The number of phase-encoding steps determines the resolution of the Y-axis for the acquired image: for example, if 128 phase-encoding steps were used there would be 128 views in the Y-axis. It is the number of phase-encoding steps which determines the total acquisition time (along with TR and the number of signal averages (NSA)).

Frequency-Encoding Gradient (X-Axis)

The frequency-encoding gradient is the last to be activated and is applied across the slice in the opposite direction to the phase-encoding gradient. The gradient produces a change in frequency across the slice causing

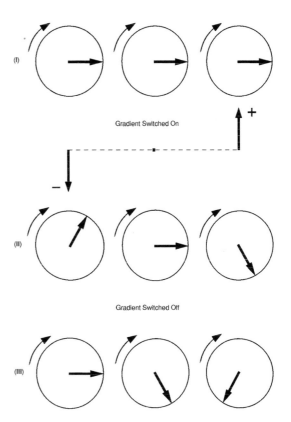

Fig. 4.3. The effect of the phase-encoding gradient. The protons precess with the same frequency but they are slightly out of phase.

Phase-Encoding Gradient (Y-Axis)

The phase-encoding gradient is activated in the time between slice excitation and signal collection (readout). Upon activation the slice undergoes a linear magnetic field change which causes the protons to precess at different frequencies in the direction that the gradient is applied. The phase-encoding gradient is then turned off and the protons begin to precess according to the strength of the magnetic field once again. As can be seen in Fig. 4.3, although the protons precess with the same frequency they are slightly out of phase.

the protons to precess according to their position along the gradient. It is the number of frequency-encoding steps which determines the resolution of the image.

It is during the application of the frequency-encoding gradient that the signal is detected and measured. The number of individual samples taken across the gradient determines the resolution of the resultant image (X-axis): for example, 256 views would give 256 voxels.

In practice, in a spin echo pulse sequence the application of the phase-encoding gradient would cause severe dephasing of the precessing protons and so in order to compensate for this a short gradient pulse (dephaser) is applied in the frequency-encoding direction before the 180° RF pulse. The 180° RF pulse inverts the phase loss caused by the dephaser and when the frequency-encoding gradient is applied complete rephasing has occurred by the time of the echo (TE), as shown in Fig. 4.4.

In Fig. 4.5 a spin echo pulse sequence is shown, indicating the timing of the three gradients described above. Most modern machines have the facility to choose the direction in which phase encoding and frequency encoding occurs.

Since phase encoding occurs many times during a scanning sequence (128 times, 256 times, etc.) then motion during this time produces artifacts in this direction. Therefore the advantage of this facility is that it allows the operator to choose the direction in which those artifacts will appear, thus preventing them from obscuring the area of interest. (Examples of this

Table 4.1. Directions of the axes for routine imaging

Plane	Frequency	Phase	Slice selection
Axial	R/L (X)	A/P (Y)	H/F (Z)
Sagittal	H/F (Z)	A/P (Y)	R/L (X)
Coronal	H/F (Z)	R/L (X)	A/P (Y)

R/L, right/left; H/F, head/foot; A/P, anterior/posterior.

will be given in Chapter 6.) The directions of the phase-encoding and frequency-encoding axes for routine imaging are shown in Table 4.1.

We now have a collection of signals received from the excited slice, composed of multiple individual frequencies each with their own relative phase shift.

K-Space

The raw image data can be thought of as existing in a matrix made up of a number of rows of data points, with each row corresponding to a single phase-encoding step and each position along that row corresponding to a different frequency (as determined by the frequency-encoding gradient). This two-dimensional matrix is known as K-space and it is the different methods of filling K-space which are utilised in fast imaging techniques.

The central portion of K-space (smallest values of phase-encoding gradients) gives rise to the intensity pattern of the image. The more peripheral portions

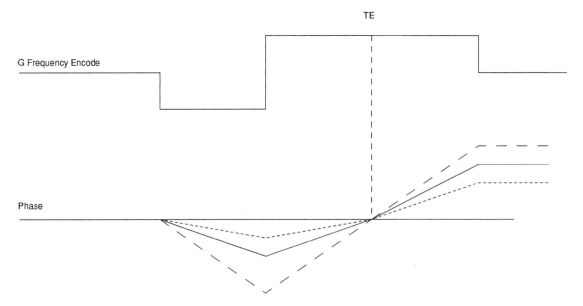

Fig. 4.4. The effect of applying the phase-encoding gradient. The 180° RF pulse inverts the phase loss.

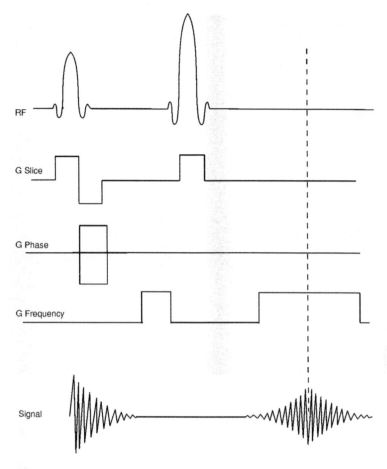

RF

G Slice

G Phase

G Frequency

Signal

Fig. 4.5. SE pulse sequence indicating the timing of the three gradients (slice, phase and frequency).

(higher phase-encoding gradient values) provide the detail of the image.

In conventional two-dimensional imaging one line of K-space is collected for each phase-encoding step during acquisition and therefore:

$$\text{Acquisition time} = \text{No. of phase-encoding steps} \times \text{NSA} \times \text{TR}$$

K-space possesses the property of conjugate symmetry, i.e. the positive phase-encoding values are symmetrical with the negative values. This can be seen in Fig. 4.6, which is a print of raw image data mapped in K-space. Half Fourier imaging utilises this fact and collects a little over half of the K-space data and computes the remaining half as a mirror image. By halving the number of phase-encoding steps in this way the total acquisition time is halved. However, there is a drawback in that the resultant images suffer from a reduction in signal-to-noise ratio (SNR) by $\sqrt{2}$, and the technique is also more susceptible to motion and magnetic field inhomogeneity.

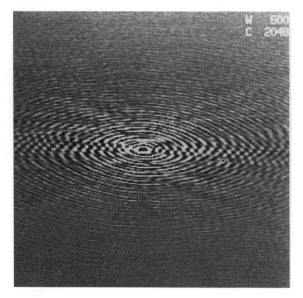

Fig. 4.6. Print of raw image data in K-space.

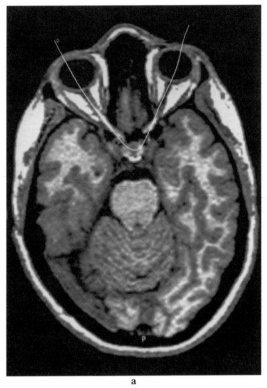 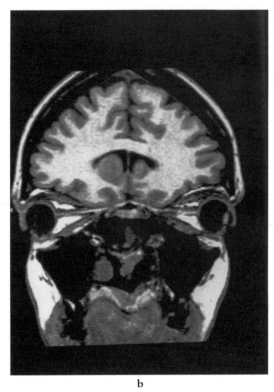

a   b

Fig. 4.7 a A single slice from a 3D data set (1 mm cubic voxels) showing the ability to reformat retrospectively in any desired plane including curvilinear reformatting. **b** The resultant reformatted image shows both optic nerves as far back as optic chiasm. (Courtesy of Picker International Ltd.)

There are other methods available of building up the raw data in K-space. Pulse sequences have been developed which use spiral, diagonal, sinusoidal and rectangular trajectories, the idea being that as much K-space as possible is built up per unit time. The ultimate in these sequences is echo planar imaging (EPI), which allows a single image to be acquired in one TR. The requirements put upon the hardware to produce rapidly oscillating gradients, together with the complex image reconstruction techniques involved, make many of these alternative (hybrid) scanning techniques suitable only for research at present.

Fourier Transformation (FT)

The signals collected during an acquisition consist of a multitude of frequency components which are superimposed to produce an interference pattern. A method has to be found which enables the breakdown of the individual phases, frequencies and amplitudes of the signals which combine to produce this pattern. The mathematical process which achieves this is performed by the computer and is called Fourier transformation (FT).

This process can be compared to the human ear and its ability to differentiate the individual instruments of an orchestra or the individual notes of a chord. FT is a very complex mathematical process and as such is beyond the scope of this text.

Three-Dimensional Fourier Transformation (3DFT)

This is achieved by three-dimensional Fourier transformation excitation of the whole imaging volume by each RF pulse and the application of phase encoding in both the slice select axis and the phase-encoding axis. This enables true contiguous slices to be obtained without loss of signal due to imperfections in slice profiles. The number of slices which the imaging volume consists of determines the number of phase-encoding steps taken along the slice select axis. Therefore doubling the number of slices would result in an increase in SNR by a factor of $\sqrt{2}$. For example, a 3 mm slice acquired from a 32 slice three-dimensional (3D) acquisition would have the same SNR as a two-dimensional slice using 32 excitations. The extra

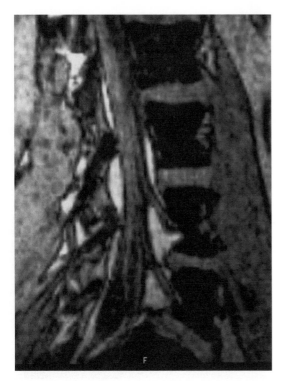

Fig. 4.8. A sagittal oblique reformat from a 3D data set of the lumbar spine showing L5 and S1 nerve roots. (Courtesy of Picker International Ltd.)

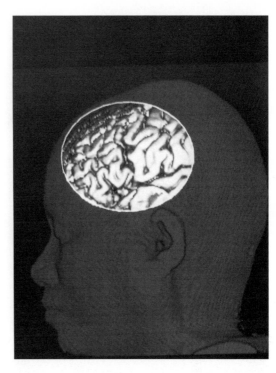

Fig. 4.9. A surface rendered image of a 3D data set of the head with a cut-away portion exposing the gyri of the brain. (Courtesy of Picker International Ltd.)

number of phase-encoding steps required during the 3D acquisition would, however, result in an increase in the scanning time. In fact for 3D acquisitions:

Total scan time = No. of slices × No. of phase-encoding views per slice × No. of excitations × TR

Once acquired, the 3D data set can be reformatted in any plane, thus allowing the single acquisition to be viewed as desired. For the images to be of high quality the voxel size should be as close to isotropic (cubic) as possible. Anisotropic voxels (rectangular cubes) cause image distortion when reformatted into their other planes. Figs. 4.7 and 4.8 are examples of reformatting and the obvious benefits of retrospective data manipulation. Another retrospective technique is surface rendering, as shown in Fig. 4.9.

5 Image Quality

High image quality is an important goal in all aspects of radiography and MRI is no exception. The MR image produced should be an exact representation of the anatomical area being imaged and therefore the quality of the image will determine the diagnostic value of the procedure. However, in MRI the decisions the radiographer has to make are different from those encountered in conventional radiography. It is therefore essential to understand the interrelationship of the different parameters and the effect of these individual parameters on the resultant image. The whole selection process is in fact a compromise, the aim being to obtain the best-quality images containing the desired information in the shortest possible time. This chapter aims to explain the relationship between the different parameters and the types of decisions to be made when selecting them.

Listed below are a number of factors which determine the intensity of the signal received; they will be covered in greater detail later in this chapter.

1. Voxel size
2. Number of signal averages
3. Pulse sequence
4. Interslice gap
5. Magnetic field strength
6. Coils
7. Centre frequency tuning
8. Receive bandwidth
9. Use of contrast media

The other factor which must be taken into consideration when referring to image quality is noise. Noise can be classified as any undesirable signal and comes from three main sources: the external environment, the patient and the system.

External noise occurs as a result of incorrect RF shielding. In the hospital environment there are a number of devices which use the same RF range as the MRI system, including fluorescent lights, electric motors, monitoring devices, televisions, elevator switching gear, computers and electric typewriters. If these external RF sources are allowed to interfere with the imager they result in noise lines appearing on and degrading the images. In most modern MRI equipment this interference is prevented from reaching the system by an RF-absorbing material (e.g. copper) that completely surrounds the magnet.

Patient thermal noise is the signal picked up by the receiver coil as a result of electrical noise generated within the tissue. Random molecular motion (Brownian motion) of the body's electrolytes within the magnetic field produces an electrical current. This random motion is dependent on body temperature, and is therefore known as "thermal noise". It is the main source of noise in the images.

System noise is always present to a certain degree. Its causes are numerous, with each electrical component within the system contributing to a greater or lesser degree. The quality of these components, the overall design and the calibration of the system have a direct influence on the amount of system noise present. In modern, properly serviced units the amount of system noise is minimal.

Other sources of undesirable signal are classed as image artifacts. Listed below are some of the artifacts commonly encountered in MRI; these will be described further in Chapter 6:

1. Cardiac motion
2. Respiratory motion
3. Flow
4. Peristalsis
5. Aliasing
6. Truncation artifact (Gibbs artifact)
7. Susceptibility
8. Chemical shift effects
9. Partial volume effects

Signal-to-Noise Ratio (SNR) and Contrast-to-Noise Ratio (CNR)

We have briefly introduced the various contributing factors determining the intensity of the MR signal as well as those factors which produce noise. The intensity of the signal within each voxel of tissue being imaged represents not only the MR signal generated by the tissue but also the noise generated within it. The amount of noise within each voxel determines how well the detected MR signal will be represented.

The signal-to-noise ratio (SNR) is a central theme in image quality and is the relationship between the signal intensity and the amount of noise detected in each voxel

Of equal importance to image quality is "image contrast", which is the difference in signal intensity of two adjacent structures. The ability to differentiate between these structures depends upon their SNR. Low contrast detection (i.e. small differences in signal) is limited by the amount of noise present.

The contrast-to-noise ratio is the ratio of the signal difference between two tissues relative to the amount of noise present

We will now discuss the factors which have a direct effect on the SNR and therefore indirectly on the CNR.

Factors Affecting SNR and CNR

Voxel Size

The most important factor determining image quality is the size of the voxel. Radiographers should be fully aware of the importance of its correct selection.

A large voxel yields a greater signal than a small voxel because of the greater number of protons available to contribute towards the image. Generally speaking, the larger the voxel the higher the SNR. This fact, however, has certain trade-offs as the larger the voxel imaged the poorer the spatial resolution due to partial volume effects which may obscure some of the smaller anatomical structures.

To achieve a greater spatial resolution the voxel size has to be reduced at the expense of a reduction in SNR, and in practice this results in grainier images.

The size of the voxel is dependent upon the following operator-definable factors:

Slice Thickness. The thicker the slice the larger the voxel size and therefore the greater SNR. (The opposite is true with a thinner slice.)

Reconstruction Matrix. The reconstruction matrix has a direct effect on the resolution of the resultant image. The matrix is determined by the number of views along both the phase-encoding and frequency-encoding axes (typically 256×256). Generally it is the number of phase-encoding views which is varied as this has a direct effect on acquisition time (128×256 would reduce acquisition time by 50% compared with 256×256). Any reduction in the number of phase-encoding views will result in a proportionate reduction in resolution along the phase-encoding axis; the SNR, however, would be increased.

A rectangular field of view is an option which allows a reduction in the number of phase-encoding steps (thus reducing acquisition time) without an increase in voxel size; the SNR, however, would be reduced using this option.

Field of View (FOV). A small FOV will reduce pixel size and therefore give good spatial resolution but at the expense of grainy images due to the reduction in signal.

SNR is proportional to FOV^2

Number of Signal Averages (NSA) or Number of Excitations (NEX)

This parameter can be expressed as the number of times the RF pulse is applied to excite the protons in a given slice of tissue. The signals detected are averaged at the end of the sequence to form the image.

Increasing the NSA results in the overall scan time being increased accordingly. For example, doubling the NSA would double the scan time. The advantage of increasing the NSA would be a direct improvement in the SNR.

SNR is proportional to $\sqrt{NSA}$

It can be seen from Fig. 5.1 that there is an obvious improvement in the SNR and also in the CNR when the NSA is increased.

The NSA can be increased to compensate for the reduction in signal from small voxels when thin-slice, high-resolution images are required. However, there is a limit to the NSA that can be selected owing to the increase in scan time, which may become impractical especially with a long TR or during T2-weighted scans.

Pulse Sequence

When considering the effect that the pulse sequence selection has on the SNR and CNR it must first be appreciated that the tissues themselves have their own

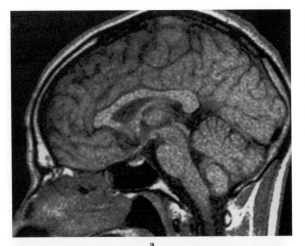

a

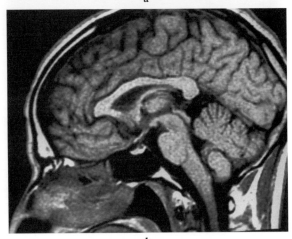

b

Fig. 5.1 a,b. Sagittal SE T1-weighted images of the brain acquired using 1 signal average (**a**) and 4 signal averages (**b**). All other imaging parameters remained constant (TR 500 ms, TE 21 ms, 5 mm slice thickness, 256 × 256 reconstruction matrix). There is an obvious improvement in the SNR which in turn leads to an improved CNR.

intrinsic properties which we have no control over. Principally these are T1, T2, proton density, chemical shift and flow.

It is the selection of the appropriate pulse sequence which enables the detection of these differences. The pulse sequences themselves have a number of different selectable parameters which control the intensity of the signal and effectively give the desired contrast in the image. These are TR, TE, TI and the flip angle, which were discussed in Chapter 3.

Interslice Gap (Spacing)

The slice profile is never rectangular (see Chapter 4) and results in tissue outside the intended slice area being excited. This has two undesirable effects. First, it reduces the spatial resolution of the image owing to the excited tissue outside the slice contributing towards the signal. Secondly, if the gap between adjacent slices is narrow then this would result in tissue at the edges of the slices being excited (cross-talk), which causes the slices to have an effective TR less than the TR set by the operator. The overall signal from the tissues would be reduced as well as the contrast.

Magnetic Field Strength

The SNR is approximately proportional to the magnetic field strength. The higher the field strength the greater the SNR.

Coils

The selection of the appropriate surface coil is of paramount importance. Localised surface coils are particularly sensitive but only to a certain depth, depending upon their design/size (Chapter 2 explains coils in more detail).

This increased sensitivity will result in an increase in SNR and therefore it is of great importance that where a high SNR and consequently high spatial resolution is required a coil is chosen the sensitivity of which fits as closely as possible the area being imaged. The trade-off, unfortunately, is that SNR decreases with increasing distance from the coil.

Centre Frequency Tuning

The procedure of centre frequency tuning matches the transmitter frequency of the system with the frequency of the protons within the patient. Precise matching is essential and any inaccuracies will result in a decrease in the SNR. Fig. 5.2 demonstrates a correct centre frequency adjustment. The procedure is carried out at the beginning of the examination and, unless the area under investigation changes, need be carried out only once. It is carried out automatically in many modern scanners.

Receive Bandwidth

The noise within the MR system is present over a wide range of frequencies. The wider the bandwidth (BW) the more noise goes into the formation of the image. In contrast a narrow bandwidth detects signal over a narrower range of frequencies and therefore proportionately less noise is present in the image, with a corresponding increase in the SNR.

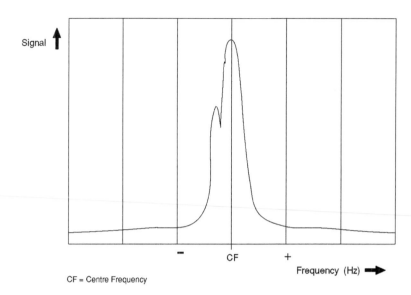

Fig. 5.2. Correct centre frequency adjustment matching the transmitter frequency of the MR system with the frequency of the protons within the patient.

SNR is inversely proportional to $\sqrt{BW}$

The trade-off which occurs in selecting a narrow bandwidth is the increase in the chemical shift artifact and limiting the selection of shorter TEs.

Use of Contrast Media

The various types of contrast media available or under evaluation have different effects on the signal intensity of the tissues. This topic will be discussed fully in Chapter 8.

The Ideal SNR

Having described the factors which influence the SNR and CNR and the way in which changing these parameters affects the SNR directly, it becomes obvious how important it is to keep these relationships in mind when prescribing a scan.

Although images with a high SNR appear pleasing to the observer and have good contrast they could probably have been acquired in a much shorter scan time, still have the same spatial resolution and information. This is because once a certain level of SNR is reached any improvements beyond this are no longer noticeable.

It is just as important not to have too low a SNR (as the image will appear grainy) as it is not to have too high a SNR

Other Factors Contributing to Image Quality

Other factors contributing to image quality are patient cooperation and the transfer of images onto hard copy.

Patient cooperation plays an important role. Scanning time may have to be minimal, at the expense of image quality, if the patient is difficult and unco-operative.

Even the best quality image can look poor if windowed incorrectly. The setting of the brightness and contrast levels (window width and level) is a very important part of the imaging process, for it is from these hard copies that the radiologist will write a report and the surgeon make a decision about whether or not to operate on the patient.

The radiographer must have a clinical knowledge of the patient in order to image the area of anatomy correctly.

Quality Assurance in MRI

Quality assurance is a very important but also very complex part of MRI. There are numerous artifacts which occur in MRI from a variety of different sources; some are present because of the inappropriate selection of pulse sequence parameters and others are caused by problems with the hardware within the system and will need the attention of the service engineer. These will be discussed in Chapter 6.

Quality assurance procedures should be carried out on a regular basis to ensure consistency of results. The most important check that can be carried out is a SNR measurement. Ideally these measurements should be taken daily for all receiver coils, but this may not be possible in practice as it is a fairly time-consuming procedure. A reasonable alternative is to take the measurements on the different receiver coils on a weekly basis with the daily SNR taken with one coil.

SNR measurements are a sensitive method of detecting a fall-off in imager performance. The measurements made do not indicate the cause of the problem, merely the effect that it has on the images. To assess the problem accurately further tests would need to be carried out. Images are obtained using a uniform cylindrical paramagnetically doped water phantom (copper sulphate solution) with a standardised SNR scanning protocol (as advised by the manufacturer). The mean pixel value within a region of interest (ROI) is the signal level. The scan is repeated twice to obtain two images at the same location and the image noise is found by subtracting one image from another. (The signal is the same in both of the images so on subtraction all that is left is the noise.) The standard deviation of the image noise within the ROI is the noise level. The head coil is usually the best coil to perform this on because of its uniformity of signal reception.

Procedure for Checking SNR

For a daily SNR check of the head coil:

1. Place the phantom in the head coil and place the coil into isocentre of magnet.

2. Select the appropriate SNR protocol.

3. Tune the scanner, i.e. centre frequency check and transmit/receive gain. Keep a record of the transmit power levels and attenuation levels.

4. Image a single axial slice twice in succession with minimum delay between scans. It is most important that all tuning values remain identical for both scans, so once tuned and set up for the first scan the tuning should not be repeated prior to the second scan.

5. Obtain the first image on the console and place a circular ROI in the centre of the phantom image.

6. Maintain the area of the circle constant throughout (e.g. 50% of the area of the phantom). Once

positioned, the computerised measurement of the signal can be obtained. Record the mean pixel value (signal level).

7. Subtract the first phantom image (compumetrically) from the second. The circular cursor is positioned centrally over the subtracted image and the computerised measurement of the standard deviation (noise level) is recorded.

8. Calculate the SNR:

$$SNR = \frac{\text{Mean pixel value} \times \sqrt{2}}{\text{Standard deviation}}$$

9. Record this reading for comparison with other SNR readings.

Because the phantom is cylindrical it is also possible to check visually the shape of the axial images produced when performing the SNR check. Ideally, if correctly positioned, the images should be a perfect circle. This is another useful indication of the accuracy of the imager.

When performing the SNR check using the surface coils care must be taken to ensure consistency of results. Their sensitivity varies with depth so it is important that the phantom is always positioned in the same way in relation to the coil. The readings should also be taken from the same place on the phantom images.

As previously mentioned the SNR check assesses overall imager performance; it is not, however, very specific at identifying the cause of a particular problem. There are further tests which can be performed using specially designed phantoms which check the many different aspects of the imager's performance. The decision as to whether or not to buy these expensive test tools depends upon the resources and goals of the institution within which the imager is sited. For example, a hospital-based imager will have completely different performance requirements from a university-based research machine.

There are a number of different phantoms commercially available which can check many of the parameters in MRI, namely: spatial uniformity, scan slice thickness and contiguity (intervals), verification of the patient alignment system, spatial resolution, geometric distortion, low-contrast sensitivity, T1 and T2 measurements, and evaluation of 3D volume reconstructions. This more specific testing is much more time consuming and requires the expertise of a suitably qualified physicist in interpreting the results. These tests can be left to the service engineer but it is good if the radiographer can perform some of them as they can play a critical role in acceptance testing and evaluating repairs/upgrades.

Other Aspects of Quality Assurance

The storage of MR data and transfer of that data onto film needs monitoring to ensure consistent results. The MR data can be stored on magnetic tape, optical laser discs or compact laser discs. This long-term storage of data allows the clearing of the system's hard disc.

Monitoring of hard copies is important for the following reasons:

1. To ensure the hard copies are of diagnostic quality.
2. To allow assessment of the sequences used with regard to diagnostic quality and potential improvements.
3. To assess the performance of the imager (laser or multi-format camera).
4. To check for any processor-produced artifacts.
5. To ensure that the correct patient data are on the film.

With regard to processor monitoring and film storage, regular departmental meetings to discuss quality assurance in its various forms allow improvements to be made.

6 Image Artifacts

The aim of this chapter is to bring to the attention of the radiographer the numerous artifacts which occur in MRI and interfere with the quality and interpretation of the images. These artifacts can obscure or create false pathology and it is therefore important to minimise or eliminate them. This can be achieved in a number of different ways.

An artifact can be described as a signal void or intensity which appears on the image and bears no resemblance to the actual anatomy of the volume being imaged.

There are several different sources of artifacts, which can be divided into the following broad categories:

1. Magnetic field artifacts
2. Hardware-related artifacts
3. Motion-related artifacts
4. Pulse sequence/data acquisition artifacts

These will be discussed in turn.

Magnetic Field Artifacts

Internal Causes of Inhomogeneities of the Main Magnetic Field

Perfect homogeneity of the magnetic field is highly desirable for good-quality undistorted images. As described in Chapter 2 any imperfections in the homogeneity of the magnetic field are compensated for by shimming. If shimming is not performed correctly the inhomogeneities will cause spatial misregistration of image data (owing to changes in the Larmor frequency) as shown in Fig. 6.1. It is therefore important in actively shimmed magnets that the shimming process is performed regularly or tests performed to check homogeneity. Resistive magnets can suffer inhomogeneities from fluctuations in their power supply. Superconductive magnets, on the other hand, produce a very stable homogeneous field.

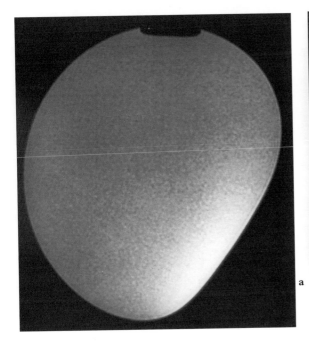

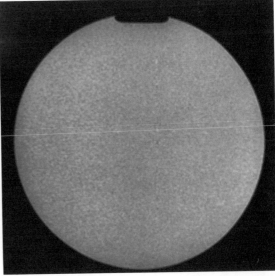

a   b

Fig. 6.1 **a** Example of an artifact produced by incorrect shimming. **b** The same image after shimming has been corrected.

Improvements in magnet design and manufacture will also minimise the degree of inhomogeneity within the magnet.

External Causes of Inhomogeneity

Metallic objects placed inside or in the immediate vicinity of the magnet affect the homogeneity by means of an effect on the magnetic lines of force. This is known as an object's magnetic susceptibility and the different types of susceptibility fall into one of three categories: ferromagnetic, paramagnetic and diamagnetic.

Ferromagnetic materials have a high magnetic susceptibility as they strongly attract the lines of magnetic force, so distorting the homogeneity of the magnetic field they are placed in.

Paramagnetic materials have a low magnetic susceptibility as they weakly attract the lines of magnetic force.

Diamagnetic materials have a very low magnetic susceptibility as they weakly repel the lines of magnetic force. This, however, has only a minimal effect on the MR signal intensities. The exception is when large changes in magnetic susceptibility are encountered (e.g. in the paranasal sinus/brain interface).

Susceptibility Artifacts

The ferromagnetic artifact is the most extreme example of a susceptibility artifact. There is distortion and signal loss within the images but whereas paramagnetic and diamagnetic susceptibility effects are only minimal, ferromagnetic effects are much more obvious.

Ferromagnetic Artifacts

Ferromagnetic artifacts have a characteristic appearance with geometric distortion, a region of decreased signal intensity and, on one side adjacent to this, a region of hyperintensity. The reason for this appearance is the method employed for spatial location in two-dimensional Fourier transformation. Ferromagnetic objects distort the linear gradient magnetic field by combining with and opposing it. This causes protons to precess at different frequencies from those expected, so causing image distortion and signal loss.

Fig. 6.2 shows an example of this type of artifact. It should be noted that although there is local distortion and signal void caused by the artifact there is still useful information in the image.

A common ferromagnetic artifact encounted in post-operative imaging results from tiny fragments of metal breaking off the surgical instruments while drilling through bone (Fig. 6.3).

Non-ferromagnetic Artifacts

Some surgical clips fall into the category of non-ferromagnetic artifacts and will produce a local signal void. The severity of this artifact depends on the shape of the clip, as this determines the clip's conductive pathway. A U-shaped clip, for example, generates less artifact than a closed loop.

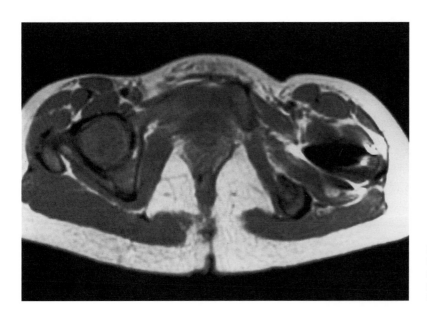

Fig. 6.2. A susceptibility artifact in the hip. Although there is a signal void and distortion locally caused by the artifact there is still useful information to be found.

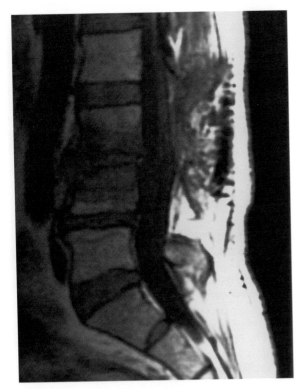

Fig. 6.3. A post-operative lumbar spine demonstrating the artifacts produced by metal fragments from the surgical instruments.

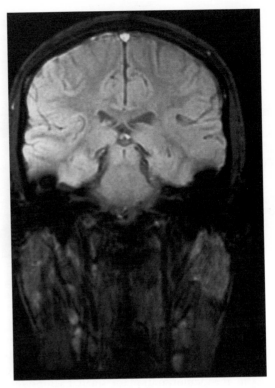

Fig. 6.4. Diamagnetic susceptibility artifact around the mastoid air cells.

Paramagnetic Artifacts

Paramagnetic substances cause shortening of the T1 and T2 times of tissues. Their presence in tissue locally enhances the return to equilibrium of the water molecules. The paramagnetic effect is observed in two main areas in MRI: (1) the MR appearances of haemorrhage and its evolution over time and (2) the use of paramagnetic contrast agents. These two topics will be discussed in detail in Chapter 11 and Chapter 8 respectively.

So by shortening the tissue's T1 relaxation time the tissue appears as a higher signal on T1-weighted images. Similarly by shortening the tissue's T2 relaxation time the tissue appears as a lower signal on T2-weighted images.

Diamagnetic Effects

Diamagnetic effects are apparent at the boundaries between tissues which have differing diamagnetic susceptibility and result in localised distortion of the magnetic field. This leads to loss of phase of spins within the voxels. This phase dispersion may cause severe reduction in the transverse magnetisation, causing loss of signal and geometric distortion.

The difference in susceptibility between air and water is in the order of 13 p.p.m. Therefore at air/soft tissue boundaries these differences in susceptibility are most apparent. Such boundaries occur in, for example, the mastoid sinuses, sphenoid sinuses and nasopharynx (Fig. 6.4).

Pulse Sequence Selection and Susceptibility Artifacts

Pulse sequence selection and susceptibility effects are much more obvious when scanning at a higher field strength, but more importantly the type of pulse sequence used to obtain the images has a bearing on the amount of susceptibility present. For example, the gradient echo pulse sequence relies on the reversal of the polarity of the gradients to rephase the transverse magnetisation and so is very dependent on the homogeneity of the magnetic field. The spin echo sequence, on the other hand, uses a 180° RF pulse to achieve rephasing of the transverse magnetisation, which means that while it is still dependent on the homogeneity of the magnetic field for spatial location, it is not so sensitive to the inhomogeneities caused by magnetic susceptibility.

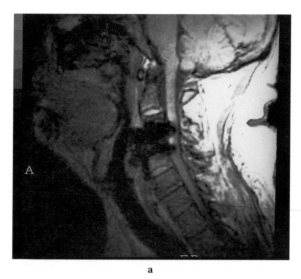
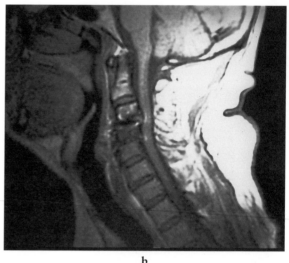

Fig. 6.5 **a** Sagittal T1-weighted gradient echo scan on a post-operative spine. **b** The same spine but this time using a spin echo pulse sequence. The susceptibility artifact is greater and causes more distortion on the gradient echo scan.

The fact that gradient echo pulse sequences are more sensitive to inhomogeneities caused by magnetic susceptibilities can on occasion be used to advantage (e.g. in the demonstration of small haemosiderin bleeds or melanin in metastatic melanoma). Calcium, too, can be demonstrated using this sequence.

The spin echo pulse sequence, however, has advantages due to its relative insensitivity to magnetic susceptibility, allowing patients with ferromagnetic particles/implants *in situ* to be scanned. As demonstrated in Fig. 6.5, the difference in the images obtained with gradient echo and spin echo pulse sequences is readily apparent, the susceptibility artifact being much more obvious and causing greater distortion on the gradient echo scan (Fig. 6.5a). The same applies to diamagnetic susceptibility. The areas of distortion and signal void around the sphenoid sinus and mastoid air cells seen on the gradient echo images (Fig. 6.4) can be minimised if not completely reduced by using a spin echo sequence.

Other Methods of Reducing Susceptibility Artifacts

In addition to the use of a spin echo sequence, there are other methods of reducing susceptibility artifacts:

1.   The use of short echo times reduces the susceptibility artifact as less time is available for the dephasing of the transverse magnetisation.
2.   The use of thin slices and the selection of small pixels reduces the amount of dephasing (partial volume effect) within the slice.

3.   The use of three-dimensional Fourier transformation volume acquisitions for gradient echo imaging is also effective for reducing dephasing within the slice.
4.   A stronger readout (frequency-encoding) gradient can decrease the artifact.

Hardware-Related Artifacts

Hardware-related artifacts are associated with the MRI machine and occur during data acquisition and image reconstruction. They are further categorised by their source, i.e. gradient artifacts, RF artifacts, computer artifacts. The digital circuits of the computer/array processor are normally very reliable and rarely fail.

Gradient-Related Artifacts

Instabilities of the magnetic field gradient can produce subtle losses in spatial resolution or, more seriously, cause ghosting in the phase-encoding direction of the image. These instabilities can be caused by thermal overload of the gradient coils and can occur when the gradients are run at a high rate with fast gradient echo techniques. They may also arise from interactions with the shim coils. Failure of a gradient amplifier or a drop-off in power would lead to image distortion.

The gradient coils also produce eddy currents, which persist in the conducting surfaces of the magnet assembly after the gradients have been switched off. They can cause the following artifacts:

1. A more rapid dephasing of transverse magnetisation (shortening T2 decay).
2. Image ghosting identical to motion-related ghosting and identifiable by its presence on phantom images.
3. Banding (zebra artifact) due to coupling of eddy currents to gradient and RF body coils in variable (multi) echo techniques.

Radiofrequency Artifacts

The RF pulses used in MRI share the same frequency range of many other RF sources, including television and radio broadcasts, computers, DC motors, electric trains, elevator switching gear and fluorescent lights to name but a few. If they interfere with the MR imager they cause an increase in image noise. The specific frequency of the external noise will determine the precise amount of interference. Frequencies the same as that of the MR imager will cause the greatest interference.

RF shielding of the magnet will prevent external RF sources from interacting with the imager and the imager's RF interacting with the external RF sources. The magnet room is shielded with copper or, more recently, aluminium to absorb and attenuate RF and thus prevent interference.

Leaks in the RF shielding can occur, particularly if the scanning door is left open or via electrical lines entering the scanner room. The latter is prevented by having RF line filters which attenuate RF in electrical lines.

Certain monitoring devices produce RF interference, such as the pulse oximeter shown in Fig. 6.6. There are, however, commercially available MRI-compatible monitoring devices which are suitably shielded.

Discrete lines or streaks seen along the frequency-encoding and/or phase-encoding axes may arise from electrical noise sources within the system due to bad components or poor electrical earthing. Such artifacts should be reported to the service engineer who will try to isolate their cause and replace or repair the defective part.

Static electricity build-up can be a source of increased noise. Certain flooring materials can cause a build-up of static, as can blankets or nylon patient gowns. Defective electric light bulbs can also cause interference.

Inhomogeneity of RF

The RF transmitter is usually tuned/calibrated around the centre slice of an acquisition, with the 90° and 180° RF pulses calibrated to produce the optimal signal. The slices remote from the centre may not be so well calibrated and this may result in RF pulses producing flip angles greater or less than 90° and 180°. The images thus produced would have a lower signal intensity from the tissues. If the 90° and 180° RF pulses are incorrectly calibrated this results in dramatic signal loss (Fig. 6.7.a) compared with the correctly tuned image (Fig. 6.7b).

Inhomogeneity of the RF due to poor coil geometry or off-centre patient positioning can cause a similar low signal intensity across the tissues. Centring

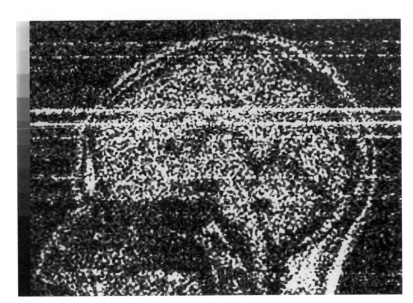

Fig. 6.6. RF interference caused by a pulse oximeter.

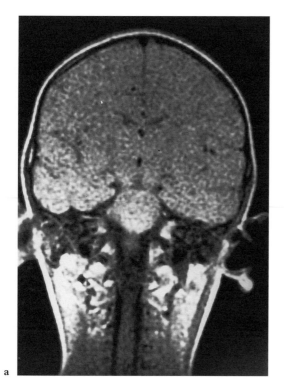 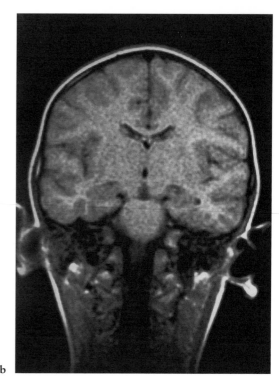

a   b

Fig. 6.7   a Result of an incorrectly calibrated 90° and 180° pulse showing signal loss. **b** Correctly tuned image.

the patient correctly can help overcome this cause of inhomogeneity.

Surface Coils

Surface coils can also generate their own artifacts due to their sensitivity extending over only a local area, according to their design. The signal drops off as the distance from the coil increases. Correct positioning of the surface coil will ensure that the area of interest is covered.

Fig. 6.8 shows the effective/sensitive range of a rectangular/quadrature, thoracic/lumbar spine surface coil. Note how the signal drops off with the distance from the coil and also how there are sharp cut-off points at the upper and lower ends of the coil.

All coils must be correctly tuned by service personnel. Incorrect impedance matching of coils to pre-amplifiers will result in the inefficient operation of the coils and at worst, noisy images or linear "zipper artifacts" occurring. Fig. 6.9a is an example of a badly tuned coil and Fig. 6.9b of a correctly tuned coil for examining the cervical spine. Fig. 6.10 is an example of a linear artifact caused by a grossly out-of-tune coil.

Physical contact between patient and coil (conducting part) causes signal loss and image distortion (Fig.

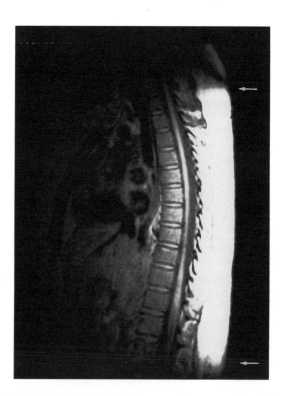

Fig. 6.8.   The effective/sensitive range of a rectangular/quadrature, thoracic/lumbar spine surface coil (*arrows* define the effective range of the coil).

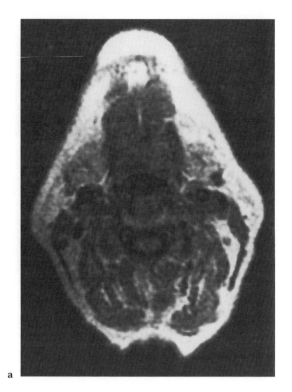

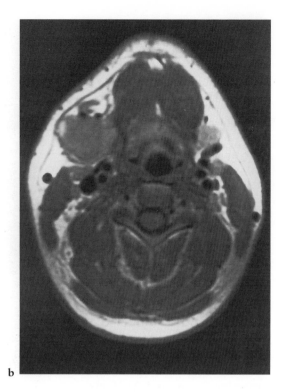

a **b**

Fig. 6.9 **a** The effect of a badly tuned coil when examining the cervical spine. **b** The image of the cervical spine with the coil correctly tuned.

6.11). It can be remedied by using a larger coil (if the area being scanned does not fit into the coil selected) or by repositioning the patient using foam pads against the body coil/surface coil to prevent electrical conduction. Alternatively a smaller field of view (FOV) could be selected so that the area of contact falls outside the FOV.

Centre Line Artifacts

Centre line artifacts can occur in the frequency-encoding or the phase-encoding direction. The artifact located centrally in the phase-encoding direction is a result of RF feed-through from transmitter to receiver because of the close proximity of one to the other. It can be reduced by alternating the phase of the RF pulses.

In the frequency-encoding direction the artifact is caused by residual transverse magnetisation in the form of free induction decay. This occurs because of slight imperfections in the shape of the 180° RF pulse. If the transverse magnetisation is not phase encoded then, if present, it will form a zipper artifact in the centre of the frequency-encoding axis.

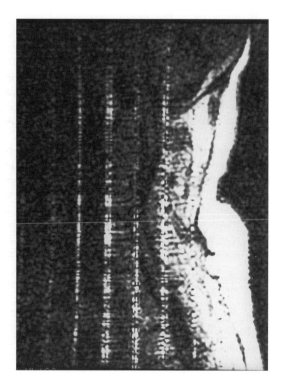

Fig. 6.10. The linear artifacts are caused by a grossly out-of-tune coil.

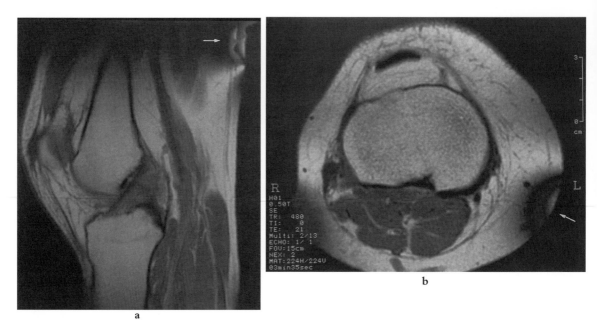

Fig. 6.11   a Sagittal SE T1-weighted image of the knee showing the typical artifact generated by surface coil contact (*arrow*). **b** The artifact in the axial plane (*arrow*).

Computer-Generated Artifacts

Once the analogue signal has been converted to a digital signal new artifacts become possible. Reconstruction errors can occur in the array processor and this can have an effect ranging from, at best, subtly changing the reconstructed image to, at worst, reducing the image to an incomprehensible pattern. Storing the raw data will allow them to be reprocessed (which may overcome the artifact encountered) or allow the service engineer to examine them and identify the fault.

Magnetic tape and optical laser discs provide most MRI units with the means of long-term data storage, but they can both be corrupted which means that data are no longer accessible.

Motion-Related Artifacts

Motion-related artifacts can be caused by periodic physiological motion (such as cardiovascular motion, cerebrospinal fluid pulsation or respiratory motion) or by voluntary (aperiodic) motion in which the patient moves. Any one of these will cause some form of image artifact – usually blurring or ghosting.

Blurring is produced by random motion of body parts during acquisition and may be caused by either a single movement or continuous motion. One conse-

quence of the motion is spatial misregistration of the image data.

Ghosting is partial outlining of image parts and is a result of periodic motion such as cardiac or respiratory motion. This occurs in the phase-encoding direction. Image ghosting can also be caused by certain hardware problems such as overheating of the cryoshield.

There are several software techniques available to help reduce or totally eliminate these artifacts, and we will now discuss some of them.

Cardiac Motion

The continuous contraction and dilation of the cardiac chambers causes obvious artifacts on the images. Software packages have been developed which allow for the synchronisation of the RF pulses to the cardiac cycle. These packages use the R wave of the patient's electrocardiogram (ECG) trace to initiate the pulse sequence. During the multi-slice sequence each slice would have data collected at a different point of the cardiac cycle. However, this point would remain consistent for each slice, e.g. slice 1 would have data collected 50 ms after the R wave for each phase-encoding step, slice 2 at 100 ms and slice 3 at 150 ms after the R wave, as shown in Fig. 6.12. Fig. 6.13a and 6.13b are examples of ungated and gated images of the chest.

The gating method described above is dependent on the consistency of the rhythm of the patient's heart

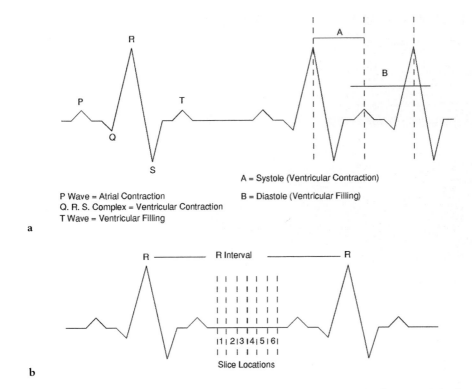

P Wave = Atrial Contraction
Q. R. S. Complex = Ventricular Contraction
T Wave = Ventricular Filling

A = Systole (Ventricular Contraction)

B = Diastole (Ventricular Filling)

a

b

Fig. 6.12   **a** The electrocardiogram (ECG) trace/pattern during the cardiac cycle.   **b** An example of sequence timing for an ECG gated study.

beat. Any arrhythmias would result in mistiming of the sequence and so produce artifacts.

The other feature of cardiac gating which should be appreciated is that the TR is dependent upon the patient's cardiac cycle and image contrast can be altered by acquiring data every other cardiac cycle (i.e. every R wave, every other R wave or every third R wave can be scanned depending on the type of contrast required). In this way T2-weighted scans are possible. The beginning of the sequence can be delayed so that imaging is possible during different phases of the cardiac cycle, i.e. during systolic or diastolic phases.

Respiratory Motion

Respiratory is another source of ghosting and blurring artifacts. The artifacts can be reduced in a number of ways.

Respiratory gating is one theoretical way to reduce the artifact. Bellows could be placed around the patient's chest which sense a change in pressure caused by the expansion of the chest wall. Alternatively a nasal sensor which picks up changes in air flow could be used. The gating would work in a similar way to cardiac gating but the disadvantage with this technique

is the long scan times that would result because of the length of the respiratory cycle (2–4 seconds). It may also prove difficult to obtain consistent gating. In general, although this technique is theoretically possible it is not used in practice in commercial systems because of prolonged scan times.

Signal Averaging

An alternative approach to eliminating ghost artifacts is to reduce their importance as a contributing factor to the overall image. Increasing the number of signal averages (NSA) increases the number of times that the image data is sampled or collected. Each voxel has its signal intensity determined by the subsequent averaging of all the different samples taken. Any artifact that has been detected on one of the samples will have a minimal overall effect as this will be averaged out by the other samples. Fig. 6.14 demonstrates this. The disadvantage with this method is that increasing the NSA increases the overall scan time proportionately. The technique of signal averaging is useful not only for respiratory motion but also for other types of periodic motion (i.e. flow).

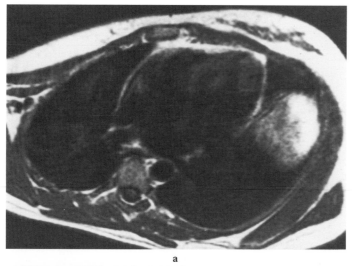

a

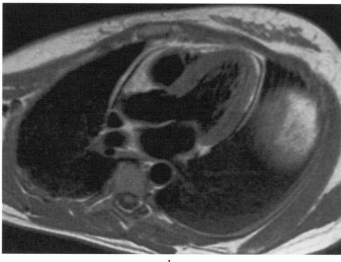

b

Fig. 6.13a,b. The effect of gating on image quality in a cardiac study. The ungated image (**a**) shows considerable motion artifacts. The gated image (**b**) is dramatically improved allowing better visualisation of the internal cardiac anatomy.

Respiratory-Ordered Phase Encoding (ROPE)

There are several different techniques available, known by the acronyms ROPE, COPE and EXORCIST. They work by rearranging the order of phase-encoding steps to correlate with respiratory motion. Each technique varies as to how this is achieved. Its use results in a slight increase in the overall scan time but the advantages far outweigh this, as shown in Fig. 6.14c.

Fat Suppression Technique

The ghosting artifact produced by respiratory motion is made more prominent because of the high signal intensity of fat which is moving with respiration. The use of the STIR sequence and other fat suppression techniques nullifies the signal from the fat and so helps to minimise the ghosting artifact, as shown in Fig. 6.15.

Breath-Holding

With the advent of fast scanning techniques such as Turbo FLASH and Fast SPGR which have scan times in the order of 1 second, a series of 15 scans through the abdomen can be completed in as many seconds and it is therefore possible to acquire these images in one breath-hold. This makes respiratory motion an artifact of the past (see Chapter 11).

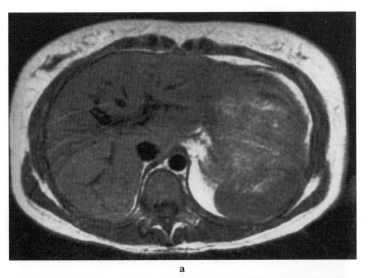

a

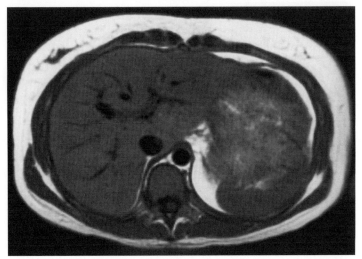

b

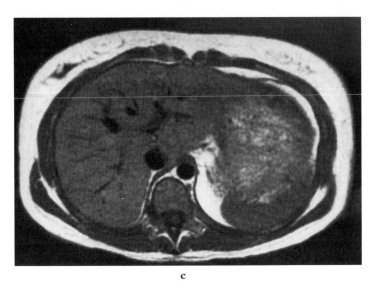

c

Fig. 6.14 **a** Axial SE T1-weighted image of the liver acquired using 2 NSA. **b** Axial SE T1-weighted image acquired using 8 NSA. All other parameters remained constant (TR 300 ms, TE 20 ms, 8 mm slice thickness, 256 × 192 reconstruction matrix using a rectangular field of view). There is an obvious reduction of the ghost artifacts. **c** Image acquired using ROPE, with all other parameters the same as in **a**. Even using 2 NSA there is definite artifact reduction.

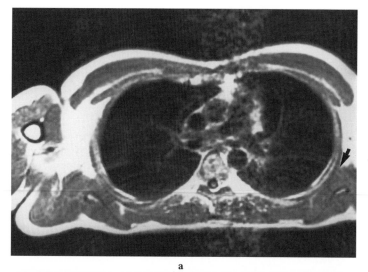

a

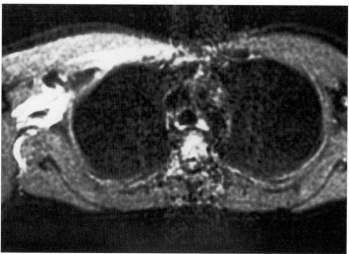

b

Fig. 6.15 **a** Axial SE T1-weighted image of the chest (TR 500 ms, TE 21 ms) showing image ghosting in the phase-encoding direction (*arrow*). These ghosts are generated by the motion of the high-signal fat in the chest wall. **b** This STIR image (TR 2000 ms, TI 100 ms, TE 30 ms) has suppressed the signal from fat and the ghost artifacts caused by respiration are removed (the vascular artifacts, however, are more pronounced with this sequence).

Other Practical Solutions to Respiratory Motion

A compression band across the abdomen will help to suppress abdominal movement during respiration. Prone positioning will also help minimise abdominal motion. This is especially useful in pelvic imaging.

Since the sensitivity of surface coils decreases with depth their use allows high-resolution images to be obtained with minimal respiratory artifact (assuming the correct positioning and selection of the coil). For example, imaging of the spine has minimal artifact from abdominal/respiratory motion as the surface coil is positioned posteriorly and is therefore insensitive to the motion of the anterior abdominal wall.

However, this is not always the case with the use of surface coils as imaging of the cervical spine would result in respiratory-related artifacts being present and

degrading the image. The effect of these artifacts can be reduced by using a software option known as "Swap Phase and Frequency" or "Gradient Rotation" which changes the phase-encoding and frequency-encoding axes.

CSF Pulsation

Cerebrospinal fluid (CSF) is produced in the choroid plexus of the ventricles. Its production (approximately 500 ml/day) causes a slow flow through the ventricular system and subarachnoid space, but superimposed on this is the pulsatile effect of the cardiac cycle. Systolic cerebral perfusion causes slight brain expansion and the ejection of CSF through the foramina of Luschka and Magendie in the fourth ventricle into the basal cisterns. The diastolic phase of the cardiac cycle results in slight brain contraction, with CSF returning into the ventricular system. This flow also occurs throughout the subarachnoid space and since this originates around the foramen magnum it is greatest in the cervical region, becoming slightly less in the thoracic region and least of all in the lumbar region.

Pulsatile CSF flow presents itself on MR images in two ways: as signal loss and ghosting. Signal loss is often seen at the aqueduct of Sylvius as a flow void. In association with flowing CSF time-of-flight (TOF) effects are present in the first and last slices of a multi-slice sequence. When a high signal intensity is seen in the first or last slice, and if this raises a diagnostic problem, the sequence could be repeated after represcription so that the slice in question appears in the middle of the imaging volume. TOF effects will be discussed in Chapter 7. Ghosting results from the CSF pulsating at velocities of up to several centimetres per second. It is most obvious in the phase-encoding direction.

There are two main ways of reducing CSF flow artifacts: cardiac/peripheral gating and flow compensation.

Cardiac/Peripheral Gating

Ghost artifacts from CSF flow can be dramatically reduced by synchronising successive pulse sequences with the ECG signal or by peripheral gating using a sensor attached to a finger.

Flow Compensation

Flow compensation, or gradient moment nulling, is a method of balancing the phase for both stationary and moving spins. These moving spins have experienced phase shifts as a result of being exposed to changing magnetic field gradients. This means that as the protons travel (flow) along a gradient then, according to the Larmor equation, their precessional frequency changes according to the other protons in their new position and this change results in intravoxel dephasing and hence signal loss.

This balancing is achieved by modifying the timing and polarity of the gradients. Fig. 6.16a–c represents three different scenarios.

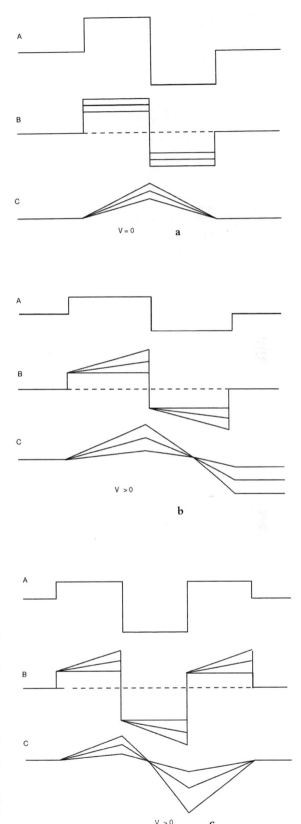

Fig. 6.16 a The effect of the applied magnetic field gradient on stationary protons. **b** The effect of the applied magnetic field gradient on protons moving with constant velocity perpendicular to the imaging plane. **c** The same as **b** but with the application of a gradient moment nulling technique. A, the gradient amplitude and polarity; B, the way in which the gradient change affects the precessional frequency; C, the phase of the protons within the slice. In all three cases rephasing of the protons is achieved.

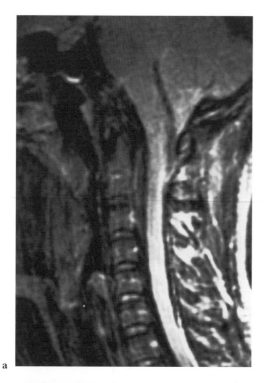

a

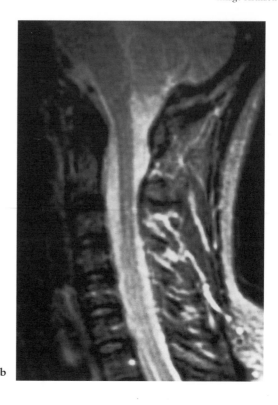

b

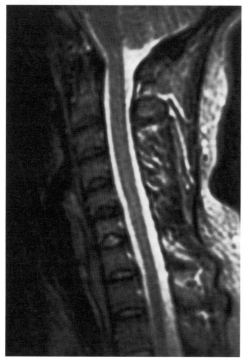

c

Fig. 6.17 **a** Sagittal SE T2-weighted image of the cervical spine (TR 2000 ms, TE 100 ms) without the use of flow compensation. **b** Sagittal SE T2-weighted image of the cervical spine (TR 2000 ms, TE 100 ms) using flow compensation. **c** Sagittal SE T2-weighted image of the cervical spine (approx. TR 2200 ms, TE 100 ms) using flow compesation and gating.

Unfortunately the trade-off for this application is an increase in the TE to allow for the additional gradient pulses. Flow compensation is most effective with in-plane flow motion and is sometimes referred to as the "bright blood" sequence because as well as rephasing the signal from CSF it also captures the signal from both slow arterial and venous blood.

Fig. 6.17a,b demonstrates the advantage of flow compensation. When used in conjunction with gating techniques it can be even more effective, as shown in Fig. 6.17c.

Blood Flow

Blood flow produces a series of artifacts which can present themselves in different ways: (1) pulsatile flow produces ghost artifacts in the phase-encoding direction, (2) flowing blood can present as a low or high signal intensity and (3) the flow signal can be misregistered on the image and appear outside the vessel in the frequency-encoding direction. All of the above artifacts can be seen in Fig. 6.18.

Methods of Reducing Blood Flow Artifacts

Cardiac/Peripheral Gating. As previously described, syn-chronising the pulse sequence with the cardiac cycle

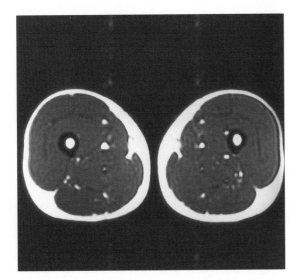

Fig. 6.18. Axial SE T1-weighted image of the thighs demonstrating the different vascular flow artifacts which can be encountered.

reduces ghosting artifacts.

Signal Averaging. Increasing the NSA (NEX) reduces the visibility of ghosting on the images. The real images gain in signal strength in proportion to the NSA. The ghost images behave more like random noise and increase in signal in proportion to the square root of the NSA. The outcome of this is a reduction in significance of ghost artifacts within the image.

The trade-off of using this technique as a method of artifact reduction is the increase in scan time: NSA is proportional to scan time, so doubling the NSA results in twice the scan time.

Swap Phase and Frequency or Gradient Rotation. Since ghost artifacts are only a problem if they appear across the area of interest and mainly in the phase-encoding direction, a solution to this is to reposition them away from the area of interest. The swap phase and frequency option allows the operator to control in which direction the artifacts will appear. This can be seen in Fig. 6.19.

Presaturation. Perhaps the most effective method of reducing vascular ghosting is by the application of presaturation pulses of RF. As the name implies, presaturation eliminates signal from tissue by nulling its magnetisation. This is achieved by adding a 90° RF pulse at the beginning of the pulse sequence, rotating the magnetisation into the transverse plane. This transverse magnetisation is then destroyed by the application of spoiler gradients, resulting in no signal during the rest of the pulse sequence.

To reduce vascular artifacts/CSF pulsation, presatu-

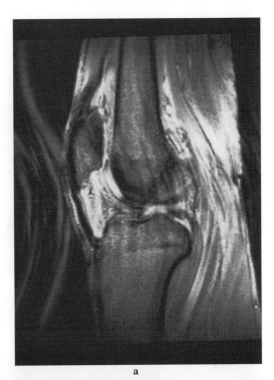

a

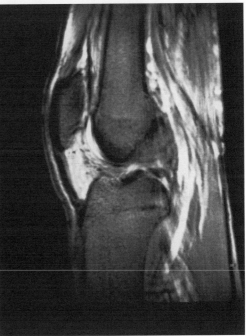

b

Fig. 6.19 **a** A gradient echo image of the knee with phase-encoding in the antero-posterior direction (*Y*-axis). Note the artifacts produced by flow within the popliteal artery and the detrimental effect that these have on the rest of the image. **b** The same gradient echo sequence with the phase-encoding direction swapped into the supero-inferior direction (*Z*-axis). The artifacts are still present within the image but they have been directed so as not to have such a detrimental effect on the image of the knee joint.

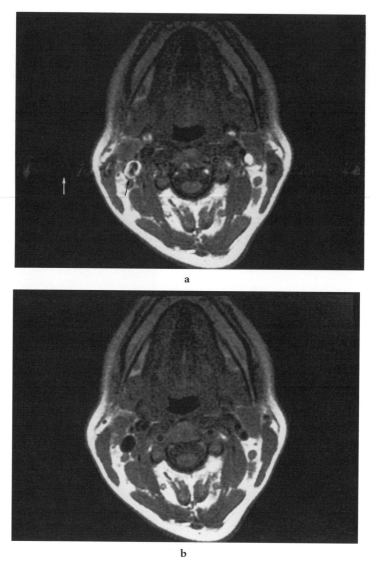

Fig. 6.20 a Axial T1-weighted image of the neck without the use of presaturation. Note the artifacts produced by the flowing arterial and venous blood (*arrows*). **b** The same sequence and slice location with presaturation applied superiorly and inferiorly. The artifacts are no longer present throughout the image and the vascular structures possess a signal void.

ration is applied (graphically or mathematically) parallel to the imaging plane resulting in minimal signal contribution from blood/CSF flowing into the volume of anatomy being imaged. This produces a signal void within the lumen of blood vessels/theca thus eliminating ghosting in the phase-encoding direction (Fig. 6.20).

Venous and arterial flow occur in opposite directions and thus it is usual to apply presaturation slabs (as they are referred to) on either side of the imaging volume to saturate the flow in either direction.

Presaturation pulses can also be utilised in other ways to prevent artifacts within the FOV and wrap-around.

Pulse Sequence/Data Acquisition Artifacts

Pulse sequence and parameter selection determine the contrast that the operator will produce in the resultant images. Their selection will also determine the amount of artifact present and its severity and type.

Other Artifacts

Inversion Recovery Bounce Point

There are two main types of reconstruction in the inversion recovery sequence: magnitude reconstruction and phase-corrected reconstruction (described in Chapter 3). The magnitude reconstruction technique is unable to recognise the polarity of the signal received. Therefore in theory the contrast of two adjacent tissues with different relaxation times could be lost if the sequence were mistimed, i.e. incorrect TI chosen.

Wraparound (Aliasing)

Wraparound, or aliasing, occurs when the FOV selected is smaller than the area of anatomy being sampled. The area outside the FOV is excited by RF and consequently the signals are detected and present themselves as artifacts overlying the tissues within the FOV. The artifacts appear as mismapped signals transposed onto the opposite side of the image and hence the term "wraparound".

The wraparound phenomenon can be explained by the Nyquist theorem, which states that periodic signals or frequencies must be sampled at least three times per cycle and, to characterise the signal correctly, at twice the highest frequency (oversampling). If the signal is sampled insufficiently (undersampling) then it is interpreted as a lower frequency and mismapped on the image. This artifact can occur in the phase-encoding or frequency-encoding direction.

Fig. 6.21 illustrates the Nyquist theorem. Applying this theory to the MR image, spatial location is achieved according to signal frequency, and therefore undersampling of the signal will produce misregistration of data on the image. This is the wraparound artifact.

The use of digital RF filters can reduce the effect of wraparound on the image in the frequency-encoding direction. This filter allows complete cut-off of signal frequency at the edges of the FOV along the frequency-encoding gradient. Also, oversampling in the frequency-encoding direction, i.e. doubling the number of views from 256 to 512, will reduce wraparound. In the same way oversampling in the phase-encoding direction will reduce wraparound artifact.

MRI systems have an imaging option available to overcome wraparound, referred to as oversampling, no

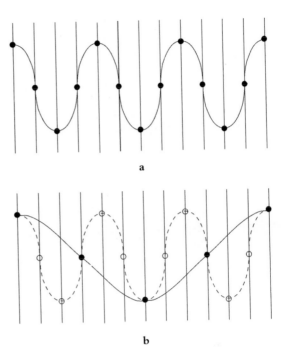

Fig. 6.21a,b. Diagram illustrating the Nyquist theorem. **a** Oversampling of the signal (at least 3 times per oscillation). **b** Undersampling resulting in incorrect frequency detection.

phase wrap, extended matrix or antialiasing. This works by doubling the FOV in the phase-encoding direction, halving the NSA and doubling the number of phase-encoding steps without any sacrifice in image quality, as shown in Fig. 6.22.

Other methods of minimising wraparound are increasing the FOV (but this is at the expense of spatial resolution) and the application of presaturation pulses outside the FOV which result in no signal being detected from those structures and therefore no wraparound.

Wraparound in the slice selection direction is not normally a problem except in three-dimensional volume acquisitions where the slices are phase encoded in both the phase-encoding and slice select directions. This results in image data from the first few slices being wrapped around onto the last few slices and vice versa. This normally results in the loss of the first and last two images within the data set. Presaturation pulses can be used to help overcome this problem also.

Truncation Artifact

The truncation artifact, also referred to as Gibbs artifact, occurs at the interfaces of tissues with high and

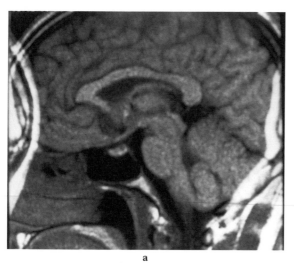 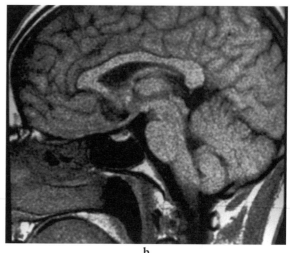

a   b

Fig. 6.22 a Sagittal SE T1-weighted image of the brain using a 17 cm FOV resulting in wraparound in the phase-encoding direction. **b** The same sequence using an antialiasing technique that removes wraparound from the image.

low signal intensities such as fat/muscle and CSF/cord.

This artifact occurs in both the frequency-encoding and phase-encoding directions and will always be present to some degree on all MR images. It is most apparent in the phase-encoding direction since the number of views in this direction is often reduced in the interests of time saving and efficiency. It normally appears as a band of low signal intensity running through a high-intensity area of the image. The fewer the number of views the more obvious the artifact becomes.

To minimise the artifact the number of phase-encoding steps can be increased until the artifact is no longer visible and the imaging time is still reasonable. Swapping the phase and the frequency directions can sometimes help to alleviate the problem also.

Clinically it is important to be able to differentiate truncation artifact from gross motion artifact and chemical shift misregistration. Ghost artifacts from gross motion reproduce themselves across the whole of the phase-encoding direction and do not fade quickly. They are not noticeably altered by changing pixel size and typically have a longer wavelength (replication interval) than that of the truncation artifact. The chemical shift artifact is encountered at water/fat interfaces and presents as bands of hypo-intensity and hyperintensity adjacent to these interfaces in the frequency-encoding direction. The truncation artifact, on the other hand, is predominantly apparent in the phase-encoding direction. Care must be taken when interpreting the truncation artifact on, for example, a sagittal T1-weighted image of the cervical spine, where the decreased signal intensity may be mistaken for a syrinx cavity.

Fig. 6.23 shows an example of a truncation artifact in the brain.

Chemical Shift Artifact

As previously described in Chapter 3, the hydrogen in fat resonates at a slightly different precessional frequency from the hydrogen in water. In fact the difference is approximately 3.5 p.p.m, with the hydrogen in fat precessing at a lower frequency. This results in a frequency difference of approximately 224 Hz at 1.5 T, 147 Hz at 1.0 T and 74 Hz at 0.5 T.

Spatial location within the image is, as described earlier, achieved by the application of gradient magnetic fields during the pulse sequence and Fourier analysis of the signals detected. The analysis of the signal assumes that the frequency shift is caused by the frequency-encoding gradient, and is not able to differentiate between that and the differences caused by chemical shift. The result of this is the misregistration of the fat-bound protons compared with the water-bound protons within the image.

The misregistration occurs in the frequency-encoding direction and since the fat-bound protons precess at a lower frequency than the water-bound protons they appear shifted to the lower-frequency side of the image (according to the applied gradient field). The result of this misregistration is an area of signal void on the image and a similar area of hyperintensity at the interfaces between fat and water. This artifact is most commonly encountered in the kidneys (Fig. 6.24), orbits, vertebral end plates and pericardium.

As previously mentioned the difference in preces-

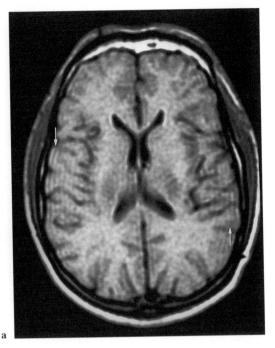
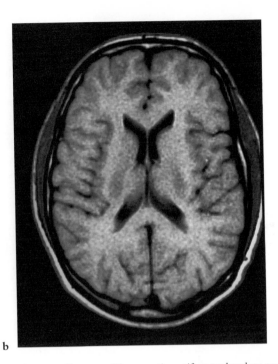

Fig. 6.23 **a** Axial SE T1-weighted image of the brain acquired with 128 phase-encoding steps. The truncation artifacts produced are easily seen (*arrows*). **b** The same sequence using an increased number of phase-encoding steps (256) results in a reduction of the truncation artifacts.

sional frequency of fat- and water-bound protons increases proportionately with field strength. The effect is therefore most obvious at higher field strengths, with a possible misregistration of as much as 3 mm!

The amount of chemical shift present is inversely proportional to the receiver bandwidth: the wider the bandwidth the smaller the chemical shift. However, the signal-to-noise ratio (SNR) is reduced according to the increase in receiver bandwidth. The operator is able to fix on the receiver bandwidth in order to compromise between the SNR and the degree of chemical shift artifact present in the image.

Chemical shift artifact presents itself in the frequency-encoding direction and by determining the direction of the frequency-encoding axis on the image the operator is, in certain instances, able to minimise the artifact. This can be useful when imaging the optic

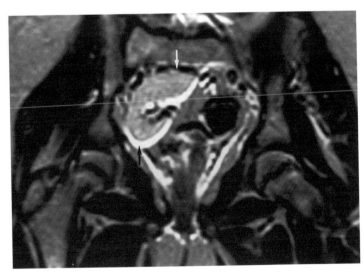

Fig. 6.24. SE T2-weighted image of the pelvis showing a pelvic kidney and chemical shift artifact (*arrows*).

nerve in the parasagittal plane, when having the frequency-encoding direction running anterior to posterior allows good visualisation of the nerve.

The differences in resonant frequencies of the water-bound and fat-bound hydrogen allow specially designed pulse sequences to saturate the fat-bound protons with RF (at a specific resonant frequency according to field strength). This occurs immediately before the main scanning sequence (90°/180° pulse pair in a spin echo sequence) and results in no signal being collected from fat-bound protons. It is particularly useful in orbit imaging.

An alternative method of separating fat and water protons is known as the Dixon technique. The 180° RF pulse of the spin echo sequence is normally applied at TE/2 to refocus the spins at TE. With the Dixon technique the timing of the 180° RF pulse is altered so as to leave fat and water either in or out of phase at TE; the subtraction or addition of these images then gives either a fat or water image.

The STIR sequence has a similar fat saturation effect as described in Chapter 3.

Cross-talk

Cross-talk results from exciting not only the slice of interest but also the adjacent slices with RF and has been discussed in Chapter 4.

The solution to the problem is to include interslice gaps, i.e. spaces between adjacent slices. For T2-weighted sequences interslice gaps of up to 50% of slice thickness are best. T1-weighted sequences require smaller gaps of 20%–30% of slice thickness. Another factor which helps reduce cross-talk is the order in which the slices are excited. Most multiple slice pulse sequences excite the odd slices and then the even slices, still using an interslice gap.

Partial Volume Effect

The partial volume effect is the result of increasing voxel size. This increases the number of anatomical structures present in the voxel and, since the signal received from these various structures is averaged in the formation of the image, the effect of this is the inability to distinguish one structure from another.

Partial volume effect has been discussed in Chapter 5 but its effects do cause misleading signals on the images and may even mask or mimic pathology. Any pathological discrepancy should be scanned in a plane perpendicular to the original plane, or thinner slices could be prescribed to produce smaller voxels and therefore reduce the effect.

7 Flow

Flow and its effects on MR images is a very complex subject. In this chapter we cover some of the basic concepts and describe the various types of flow that are likely to be encountered.

Flow phenomena are mainly associated with blood (haemodynamics), but when considering flow effects it should be remembered that the same principles apply also to cerebrospinal fluid flow.

Haemodynamics

Initially we will consider blood as a simple fluid. If the blood flow along a vessel were constant then the velocity profile of the blood within the vessel would be laminar with a parabolic profile. Fig. 7.1 demonstrates such a profile. The reason for this profile is the frictional forces against the walls of the vessel and also between the different components of the blood. The flow would be slowest against the wall of the vessel and fastest in the centre of the vessel.

Blood, however, does not behave like a simple fluid. Its viscosity is dependent upon velocity, with viscosity being high when it is flowing slowly and vice versa.

Laminar flow occurs predominantly in small-caliber vessels. In the larger-caliber vessels vascular pulsations and vessel size cause a "plug"-shaped rather than a parabolic velocity profile. This plug profile is so called because of the uniform velocity across the vessel, and is demonstrated in Fig. 7.2.

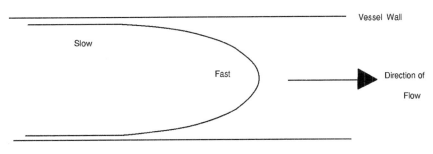

Fig. 7.1. Parabolic laminar flow in a vessel.

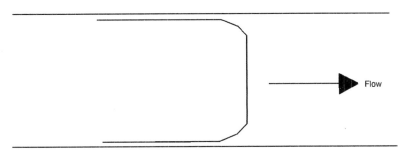

Fig. 7.2. Plug velocity in a vessel.

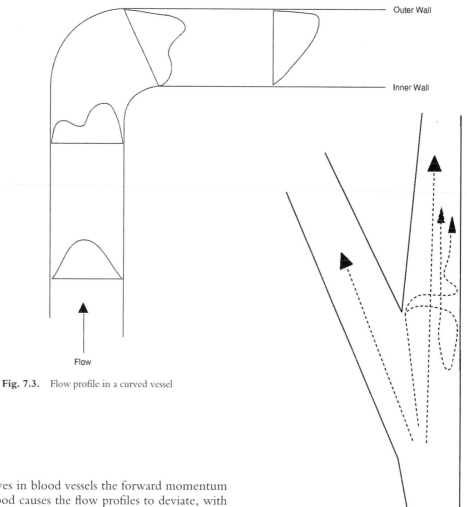

Fig. 7.3. Flow profile in a curved vessel

Fig. 7.4. Flow pattern at a vessel bifurcation.

At curves in blood vessels the forward momentum of the blood causes the flow profiles to deviate, with the faster flow occurring towards the outer wall of the vessel. Fig. 7.3 shows the flow profile in a curved vessel.

Flow patterns change too at vascular bifurcations, with secondary flow patterns developing and even retrograde flow occurring on the vessel wall opposite the bifurcation (e.g. carotid bulb). Fig. 7.4 demonstrates the flow pattern at a vessel bifurcation.

The other important flow phenomenon encountered is that of turbulence. Turbulence is defined as chaotic flow with randomly fluctuating velocity components.

At normal blood flow velocities laminar flow is predominant. Under certain circumstances, for example an area of stenosis, the blood velocity increases and exceeds a critical threshold so that turbulence is encountered. Fig. 7.5 shows turbulent flow distal to an area of vascular stenosis. (Turbulent flow should not be confused with the localised slowly swirling or stagnant flow known as vortex flow which occurs immediately distal to the stenosis.)

Appearance of Flow on MR Images

Having very briefly described the different aspects of haemodynamics we will now consider the appearance of flow on MR images.

On conventional spin echo pulse sequences flowing blood usually appears either as signal void (fast-flowing arterial blood) or with a high/intermediate signal (slowly flowing venous blood). This is a very simplistic way of looking at the subject because there are a number of other factors which influence the appearance of blood flow on the images.

The appearances can be attributed to one of four main categories of effect: (1) time of flight (TOF) effects, (2) phase effects, (3) turbulence and (4) pseudogating.

Time of Flight (TOF) Effects

TOF refers to the fact that blood will continue to flow through the slice during acquisition and, according to its speed of flow, will be represented by a high or low signal.

Slow-flowing blood will produce an increased intraluminal signal due to unsaturated blood entering the slice and being available to produce maximum signal. The signal produced is actually greater than that of stagnant blood and is referred to as flow-related enhancement. This effect is most prominent using single slice techniques or in the first or last few slices of a multi-slice technique.

Fast-flowing blood, however, due to the same phenomenon, will travel at such a speed that it will exit the slice before a signal is detected. It will therefore produce a signal void known as high-velocity signal loss or the washout effect.

Flow-Related Enhancement

Flow-related enhancement occurs mainly in vessels with slow flow and is most obvious in those vessels which are perpendicular to the imaging plane and in the same direction as the slice select gradient.

As described previously, repeated RF excitation of tissue results in partial saturation of that tissue (depending on the TR and T1 of the tissue) and the degree of saturation determines how much signal the tissue will produce. Unsaturated protons produce a higher signal than saturated protons. Let us now consider the effects of unsaturated protons in flowing blood entering the imaging slice. The blood protons would be excited by the RF along with the rest of the slice and, being unsaturated, would produce a high-intensity signal. These blood protons would quickly become saturated after entering the slice, but because they are continually being replaced by unsaturated blood there would always be a high signal detected compared with that from the stationary, partially saturated tissue.

Flow-related enhancement is most pronounced in single slice imaging or in the outer slices of multi-slice imaging. In multi-slice techniques, as the blood penetrates other deeper slices it becomes more saturated as it is subjected to further RF pulses for each excited slice that it enters.

Flow-related enhancement is greater when short TR times are used and also when tissues with a long T1 relaxation time are imaged within the slice.

High-Velocity Signal Loss or the Washout Effect

In a spin echo pulse sequence a 90° RF pulse is applied followed by 180° pulse. If blood is moving rapidly within the selected slice some of the blood will exit the slice before receiving both RF pulses. This means that the protons in this moving blood receive a 90° pulse then leave the slice before receiving the 180° RF pulse and so are flipped only 90°. In the next slice selection they will encounter another 90° RF pulse and that will result in a total flip of 180°. Vectors in a 180° position do not give a signal and therefore rapidly moving blood will be represented by a signal void.

The greater the velocity of the blood the more

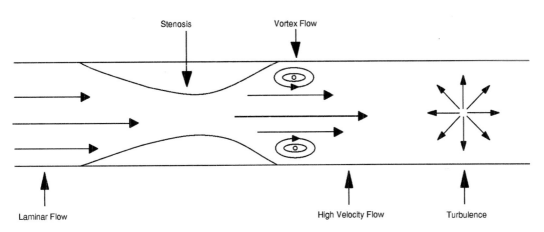

Fig. 7.5. Turbulent flow distal to an area of stenosis.

unsaturated it remains, as it flows through the slice too quickly to experience the RF pulses and become saturated.

Gradient Echo Sequences

The type of pulse sequence selected has an effect on the intensity of the signal from the flowing blood and a gradient echo pulse sequence is more sensitive to flow-related enhancement. This is because gradient reversal is used to rephase protons instead of the 180° RF pulse used in a spin echo pulse sequence and, since TE is shorter, the blood does not get a chance to move out of the slice before the signal is detected. This results in an increase in the TOF effect, i.e. an increase in signal.

Since gradient echo sequences are acquired quicker (by the use of small flip angles and short TE times) than spin echo sequences they are ideal for imaging blood flow.

Phase Effects (Even and Odd Echo Effects)

Phase effects can be divided into reversible (odd echo dephasing and even echo rephasing) and irreversible (turbulence) effects.

Odd Echo Dephasing and Even Echo Rephasing

Odd echo dephasing and even echo rephasing occurs with laminar flow in a vessel as there is dephasing of the blood protons. The protons in the imaging vol- ume are not all moving at the same speed through the magnetic field gradients and are therefore precessing at different frequencies. They are thus out of phase at the time of echo (TE), so producing a signal loss. In a multi-echo sequence all the odd echoes will, due to dephasing, have a signal loss, while the even echoes will have increased signal intensity. If laminar flow is constant and continues until a second echo is acquired the dephasing seen on the first echo will be rephased at the second and subsequent even echoes.

Turbulence

As previously described, turbulence occurs in areas distal to stenosis and is random in motion. This causes a dephasing of the blood protons as they move through the magnetic gradients and produces a signal loss.

Pseudogating

Arterial flow is pulsatile and related to the cardiac cycle. During the systolic phase of the cardiac cycle arterial blood is moving rapidly; during the diastolic phase, however, blood is moving very slowly if at all.

It is possible, depending on the patient's R-R interval, to synchronise the patient's cardiac cycle to the console-set TR. For example, a heart rate of 60 beats per minute has an R-R interval of 1000 ms. If the console-set TR were 1000 ms then images would be acquired as though gated to the cardiac cycle.

The images acquired during systole would have a signal void within the lumen of arteries, but the images acquired during diastole would have high sig-

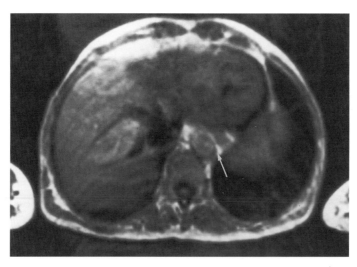

Fig. 7.6.   Example of pseudogating showing signal within the aorta (*arrow*).

nal intensity within the lumen. This can be seen in the aorta on occasions. Fig. 7.6 shows an example of pseudogating.

Magnetic Resonance Angiography (MRA)

The flow phenomena discussed above have led to the development of pulse sequences specifically designed to enhance these effects and enable the visualisation of blood vessels. These pulse sequences, used in conjunction with specialised computer-controlled processing techniques, provide the ability to perform MRA and almost all manufacturers now supply software options allowing its implementation.

The different methods employed to produce MRA images are: two-dimensional Fourier transformation (2DFT) and three-dimensional Fourier transformation (3DFT) time of flight (TOF), 2DFT and 3DFT phase contrast (PC) and 2DFT cine angiography.

2DFT Time of Flight (TOF)

The 2DFT TOF method relies on flow-related enhancement to differentiate moving spins from stationary spins as previously described. A modified gradient echo pulse sequence is used as it is most sensitive to flow. Blood flowing into the slice is fully magnetised (unsaturated) and gives off a higher signal than the surrounding (saturated) tissues.

When blood is flowing perpendicular to the slice, maximum flow-related enhancement is achieved. If a blood vessel runs parallel along the slice the blood flowing within the vessel, being exposed to multiple RF pulses, soon becomes saturated, giving off little or no signal. In a similar manner slow-flowing venous blood may become saturated within the imaging slice and so appear with a lower signal intensity (compared with faster-flowing arterial blood).

Operator-Controlled Parameters

There are several operator-controlled parameters which affect the appearance of blood. These are: TR, flip angle and slice thickness.

TR. The TR must be short in relation to the T1 of the tissues (i.e. 40–60 ms) in order to achieve signal suppression of the stationary tissues.

Flip Angle. The flip angle selected should be large enough to saturate stationary tissue but small enough not to saturate the blood. A 40°–60° flip angle will give the desired result.

Slice Thickness. The thinnest slice possible will give the greatest inflow enhancement and reduce intravoxel dephasing.

Physiological Parameters.

There are several physiological parameters which also affect the appearance of blood. These are: T1 of blood, flow rate and direction of flow.

The T1 of blood is relatively long and when flowing slowly blood will soon become saturated by the repeated RF excitations. This results in signal loss. Obviously in fast-flowing blood the opposite occurs, with maximum signal being received from it. One way to increase the signal from slow-flowing blood is to shorten its T1 using an intravenous contrast agent (e.g. gadolinium-DTPA).

Presaturation Pulses

It may be desirable to obtain angiographic images of just the arteries. This can be achieved by the careful selection and placement of presaturation pulses above or below the imaging plane according to the direction of flow. The presaturation pulse saturates the flowing blood before it enters the imaging plane, so nulling the flow-related enhancement in that direction.

This technique is particularly useful when imaging the carotid vessels where the jugular vein can overlie them. The placement of a presaturation pulse above the imaging slice allows visualisation of the carotid arteries and so reduces the risk of misinterpreting the image. The opposite can apply if the jugular veins are to be imaged, when placing a presaturation pulse inferiorly would null the arterial signal.

The neck is not the only region where this technique can be utilised. It can be used, for example, in imaging the venous supply of the pelvis by applying a superior presaturation slab.

Clinical Applications

The 2DFT TOF technique can be used for a wide range of studies. These include evaluation of the carotid bifurcation (Fig. 7.7), evaluation of the pelvic veins for deep vein thrombosis, evaluation of the lower extremities, investigation of suspected basilar

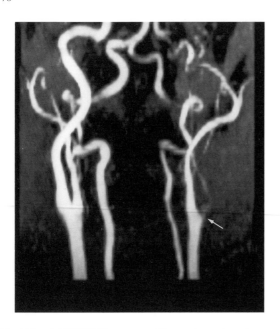

Fig. 7.7. A 2DFT TOF sequence with a maximum intensity projection (MIP; coronal view) demonstrating the arterial blood flow in the neck and showing partial occlusion of the internal carotid artery (*arrow*). (Courtesy of Philips Medical Systems.)

artery occlusion and suspected intracranial venous thrombosis, and cortical venous mapping.

Limitations

There are several trade-offs when using 2DFT TOF which may cause misleading results. First, it is relatively insensitive to in-plane blood flow, which may simulate vascular occlusion. It is sensitive, however, to patient motion, which may result in misregistration of the image. A stenosis may appear more severe than it actually is due to turbulent flow. Also, simulated flow-related enhancement can result from short T1 substances such as methaemoglobin present in subacute haematomas. Finally, the use of thin slices, small FOV and flow compensation puts a limit on the TE available.

Advantages

The advantages of 2DFT TOF are that it is sensitive to slow flow states, there are minimal saturation effects for normal flow velocities, and short acquisition times (5–7 minutes) are possible.

3DFT Time of Flight (TOF)

The 3DFT TOF technique acquires a whole three-dimensional volume or slab of tissue with saturation of the stationary tissue and flow-related enhancement from blood entering the slab.

Compared with 2DFT TOF angiography there are several advantages of 3DFT TOF angiography, including the ability to use very thin slices, an increase in the SNR, and reduced sensitivity to turbulence and pulsation.

Operator-Controlled Parameters

There are several operator-controlled parameters available, including: TR, TE, flip angle, slice thickness, matrix, flow velocity, selection of imaging volume and flow compensation.

TR. As with two-dimensional sequences a short TR (i.e. 40 ms) will give maximum saturation of the stationary tissue. If TR is reduced to less than 40 ms the spins flowing through the imaging volume become saturated which results in a loss of signal intensity in the vessel.

TE. TE should be kept as short as possible to reduce motion phase errors.

Flip Angle. Flip angle has a very influential effect on the signal intensity of the vessels. A flip angle of 15°–20° is usually successful for visualising the larger arterial structures as well as the peripheral vessels. If the flip angle is increased the stationary tissue becomes more saturated also, as do the smaller vessels with slower flow which will be seen with less signal intensity. Flip angles of more than 40° result in the arterial flow becoming saturated and therefore a reduction in signal intensity in the vessel. It is worth remembering here that the flip angle used is produced by a certain amount of RF power: the greater the flip angle the greater the RF power required to produce it.

Slice Thickness. 3D TOF is capable of very thin slices which will minimise signal loss due to phase dispersion within the voxel. The trade-off for this is that it also reduces the SNR and the volume which can be covered. A slice thickness of 0.7–1.0 mm is usually used.

Matrix. A matrix of 128, 192 or 256 is used depending on the desired resolution required and the imaging time available. One NSA can be used to keep imaging time down. A combination of matrix and slice thickness should ensure isotropic (cubic) voxels, allowing

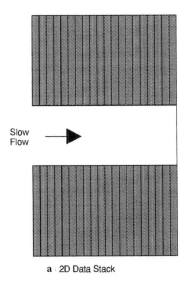

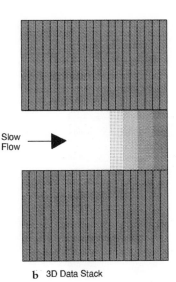

a 2D Data Stack　　　　　　　　　**b** 3D Data Stack

Fig. 7.8 a,b. The degree of saturation which occurs within slow-flowing blood vessels in a 2DFT TOF (**a**) and a 3DFT TOF (**b**) angiogram. This would result in signal loss in the vessel, the further into the volume it gets.

more accurate visualisation of vessels when projected into different planes. The smaller the voxel size the less chance there is of intravoxel dephasing.

Flow Velocity. The velocity of the blood also plays an important role in the intensity of the signal. Slow-flowing blood becomes saturated as it moves through the imaging volume and therefore signal intensity decreases, as in the case of venous thrombosis, vascular occlusion and some aneurysms. Fig. 7.8 demonstrates the proportion of saturation within a blood vessel using 2D and 3D TOF techniques.

Fast-flowing blood is fully magnetised and leaves the imaging volume between RF pulses, creating optimal signal enhancement.

Imaging Volume. The plane selected will decide the most sensitive direction of flow (with the most sensitive flow being perpendicular to the imaging plane). This must be taken into account when considering the area being examined in order to try to show the vessels of interest most effectively. For example, to demonstrate the circle of Willis an axial volume would be acquired; this requires only a small imaging volume and so reduces imaging time. It also means that the fast-flowing fully magnetised protons arrive unsaturated at the circle of Willis. In contrast, either sagittal or coronal volumes would result in the blood from the carotid arteries being saturated prior to entering the circle of Willis.

Flow Compensation. The use of flow compensation reduces phase dispersion caused by flow and maximises the intravascular signals. This, however, usually

requires a longer TE than is desirable and cannot compensate for less constant flow changes (e.g. acceleration at curves in arterial vessels, resulting in signal loss).

Clinical Applications

The clinical applications of 3DFT TOF include the visualisation of arteriovenous malformations (demonstration of arterial supply and nidus and flow aneurysms: Fig. 7.9), aneurysms, venous angiomas (using contrast media), carotid occlusion (Fig. 7.10), thoracic vessels and abdominal vessels.

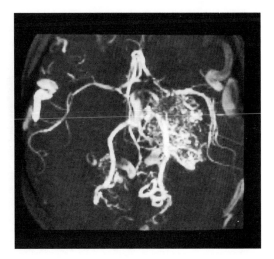

Fig. 7.9. A 3DFT TOF sequence with MIP (axial view of cranial vessels) demonstrating a large arteriovenous malformation. (Courtesy of Siemens.)

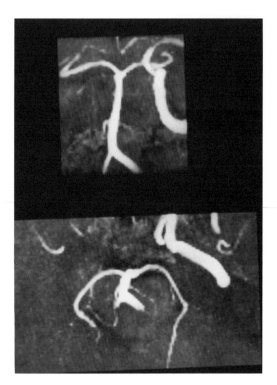

Fig. 7.10. A 3DFT TOF sequence with MIP (Coronal and axial projections of the circle of Willis) demonstrating absence of signal in the left internal carotid artery, implying occlission.(Courtesy of Siemens)

Limitations

A limitation of 3DFT TOF is its insensitivity to slow flow, which means that venous flow cannot be well demonstrated under normal circumstances. However, with the use of T1-shortening contrast agents the venous anatomy can be better visualised. As with 2DFT TOF, materials with a short T1 (e.g. methaemoglobin) appear bright on the images.

Advantages

The advantages of 3DFT TOF are its relatively short scan times, sensitivity to fast and intermediate flow, high spatial resolution and high SNR.

Magnetisation Transfer Contrast Angiography

Magnetisation transfer contrast (MTC) can be used in conjunction with either two- or three-dimensional TOF sequences and has been shown to improve small vessel detail significantly as it improves background noise suppression (Fig. 7.11).

2DFT Phase Contrast (PC)

Phase contrast angiography uses velocity-induced phase shifts to distinguish between flowing blood and surrounding tissue.

A slice of tissue is excited by the application of an RF pulse followed by two equal but opposite "bipolar" gradients. Protons moving along the direction of the bipolar gradients experience phase shifts between the application of the two gradients, while the stationary tissue does not. PC angiography is based on these phase shifts.

The size of the phase shifts depend upon how far the flowing protons have travelled between the application of the bipolar gradient pulses. Faster-flowing protons will demonstrate greater phase shifts. When the amplitude of the bipolar gradient pair is inverted a second acquisition is made and this causes a phase shift in the flowing protons opposite to the first.

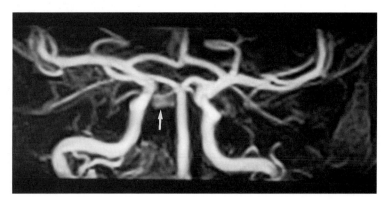

Fig. 7.11. MIP of a 3DFT TOF sequence (coronal projection of the circle of Willis) with an MTC pulse producing improved background suppression, demonstrating an aneurysm arising from the superior cerebellar artery (*arrow*). (Courtesy of Picker International Ltd.)

Using a special reconstruction the first phase shift is subtracted from the second to suppress the background signal from the stationary tissue. The information remaining is the signal that is different in the two acquisitions, i.e. the intravascular signal from the moving blood.

Operator-Controlled Parameters

There are several operator-controlled parameters which influence the final image. These are: TR, flip angle, slice thickness, matrix, velocity encoding and PC flow compensation.

TR. Since PC angiograms are much less sensitive to saturation effects a short TR is used (in the region of 25–30 ms).

Flip Angle. A large flip angle (60°–90°) would result in saturation of the smaller, slower-flowing vessels and hence loss of signal. Smaller flip angles (15°–30°) reduce the saturation effects and are therefore more desirable for demonstrating small vessels.

Slice Thickness. The thinner the slice the less complex the flow within that slice and hence the lower the signal loss due to phase dispersion.

Matrix. The matrix determines the overall dimension of the voxel and therefore the degree of phase dispersion within the voxel. Smaller voxels are more desirable but, as well as prolonging scan time, there is also the possibility (particularly in systems with low and mid strength fields) that there is insufficient signal to acquire diagnostic images.

Velocity Encoding. The velocity-encoding value determines the amplitude of the flow-encoding gradient. If this is set too low, for example, then high-velocity flow will appear as a low signal, due to aliasing.

PC Flow Compensation. This can be applied in a slightly modified form to enhance vascular signal.

Clinical Applications

The clinical applications of 2DFT PC angiography include investigation of occlusion of the basilar artery, dural sinuses, intracranial venous structures, sagittal sinus, arteriovenous malformations (Fig. 7.12), slow-flow components of large aneurysms and the portal venous system. It can also be used as a pilot study prior to the main 3DFT PC study to ensure that correct velocity encoding is applied.

Limitations

A limitation of 2DFT PC is the large voxel size, which results in increased intravoxel dephasing.

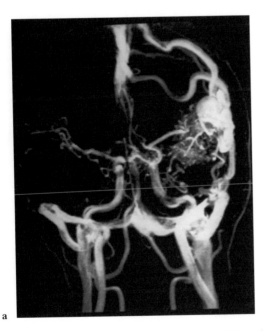
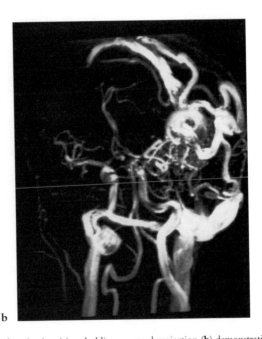

a b

Fig. 7.12 a,b. A 3DFT phase contrast sequence with MIP in the coronal projection (**a**) and oblique coronal projection (**b**) demonstrating a large cranial arteriovenous malformation. (Courtesy of Philips Medical Systems.)

Advantages

The advantages of 2DFT PC are that images can be acquired in a few minutes, there is excellent suppression of stationary tissue, it is extremely sensitive to slow flow (so it is good for venous and arterial imaging) and to directional flow, and it is able to generate magnitude and phase (directional) images.

3DFT Phase Contrast (PC)

In 3DFT PC data are acquired with additional phase encoding in the slice select plane/direction, in a similar manner to 3DFT TOF. The three-dimensional data set has all the features of the 2DFT PC image but with the additional benefit of having very small voxels.

Data are usually acquired from the three flow-encoding directions and then combined to produce the final images. These can be viewed individually or in compumetric projections.

Factors Affecting Contrast

The factors that affect contrast in 3DFT PC are flow direction, velocity encoding, phase dispersion and flip angle.

Flow Direction. The bipolar flow-encoding gradients have to be applied in every direction in which flow data are sought. Every time the gradients are reapplied the scan time is increased. With simple unidirectional flow (e.g. in the carotid vessels) only one direction of flow encoding is required. Where there is more complex multi-directional flow (e.g. in the circle of Willis), however, flow encoding must take place in all three directions.

Velocity Encoding. Selection of the highest velocity likely to be encountered within the vessel of interest is very important in order that the amplitude of the bipolar flow-encoding gradient can be adjusted to allow imaging of all velocities up to and including the velocity set. If the velocity encoding is set too low then peak velocities higher than the level set will be aliased and appear as low signal intensities in the centre of the vessel.

Phase Dispersion. Dispersion of velocities within blood vessels results in variations of phase shifts, with the overall signal from that vessel representing the average velocity. If flow is complex or turbulent the dispersion of phase shifts may cause signal loss or even zero signal. This can be greatly reduced by obtaining thin

section images (as in three-dimensional volume imaging) of the vessels in cross-section rather than in profile.

Flip Angle. As with the TOF imaging, increasing the flip angle increases the saturation of the smaller peripheral vessels. Typically in cranial imaging flip angles of 15°–30° are used without loss of signal due to saturation effects.

Quantitative Applications

If the raw data from phase contrast angiography are post-processed there is the potential for velocity measurements. Fig. 7.13 shows how this is possible.

The phase images are sensitive to flow in different directions, which can have useful applications. Figs. 7.14 and 7.15 are examples of phase images.

Clinical Applications

The clinical applications of 3DFT PC include evaluation of aneurysms and arteriovenous malformations, demonstration of venous thrombosis, imaging large volumes and evaluation of traumatic vascular injury.

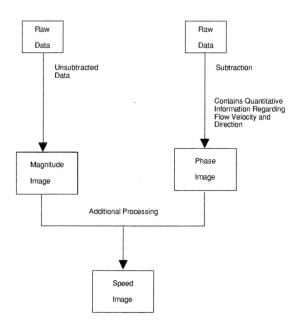

Fig. 7.13. Flow diagram showing the calculation of magnitude, phase and speed images from a phase contrast angiographic data set.

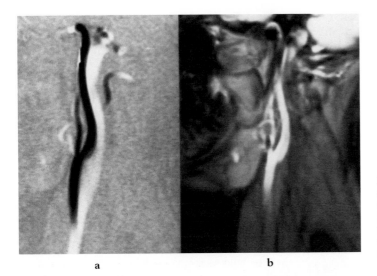

a   b

Fig. 7.14 a,b. A 3DFT phase contrast sequence demonstrating the neck vessels (sagittal). **a** The subtracted image showing the different flow directions (*white*, caudal [venous] flow in the internal jugular vein; *black*, cranial [arterial] flow in the carotid artery). **b** An unsubtracted image from the original data set. (Courtesy of IGE Medical Systems.)

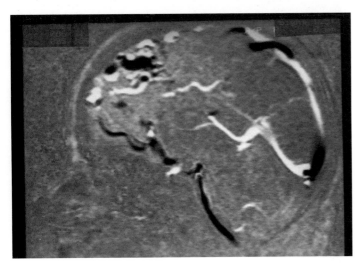

Fig. 7.15. A 3DFT phase contrast image of cranial vessels showing an arteriovenous malformation and the direction of flow into and out of the lesion (*black*, cranial flow; *white*, caudal flow).

Limitations

The main limitation of 3DFT PC is its relatively long imaging times. It is slightly more sensitive than TOF techniques to signal loss from turbulence.

Advantages

The advantages of 3DFT PC are its reduced intravoxel dephasing, good background suppression, improved SNR compared with 2DFT PC, ability to encode for different velocities of flow, minimal saturation effects over large volumes, ability to image venous and arterial structures, and its ability to generate magnitude and phase images and to measure velocity. It is superior to TOF methods in regions of slow flow and in tortuous vessels.

Post-processing of MRA Data

The series of slices acquired by sequential two- or three-dimensional angiography are processed by a method known as the maximum intensity projection (MIP) ray tracing technique.

The technique uses a straight line or ray which is projected through the acquired slices along a selected plane. The ray represents a single pixel and each pixel corresponds to the intensity of the brightest voxel intersected by the ray. A series of rays is projected through the volume, each representing the intensity of one pixel (the brightest) in the plane. Since the brightest voxel represents flowing blood, only vascular structures are displayed in the resultant image.

Two- or three-dimensional images may be processed in this way although it is most suitable in imaging rapidly flowing blood because slow-flowing blood will be more saturated and so is difficult to distinguish from stationary tissue. This means the MIP algorithm is unable to select the vessels in the final image.

The process may be repeated in other planes and the collection of projected images viewed as a cine loop to give the appearance of rotation and depth, representing a three-dimensional image of the vascular structures.

The disadvantages of post-processing are a slight decrease in vessel diameter that may cause inaccurate estimation of stenosis, and the fact that overlapped vessels are presented as a single vessel.

2DFT Cine Angiography

2DFT cine angiography is a gradient echo technique that acquires multiple images at the same slice location during different stages of the cardiac cycle. This technique, used in conjunction with flow compensation, produces a bright signal from the continuous inflow of fresh blood. Turbulent, complex flow, however, produces a low signal intensity due to phase dispersion. This effect can be used to assess cardiac valve regurgitation.

Measurement of Flow

MRI can be used to measure flow velocity. The two main methods are presaturation bolus tracking and phase shift effects (zebra stripes). The theory behind these techniques is beyond the scope of this text.

8 MR Contrast Agents

In this chapter we will cover the different types of contrast media available and their applications in MRI.

The excellent tissue differentiation observed in the earliest MR images provided the clinician with so much information that the need for a contrast agent seemed unlikely. However, as the technique progressed, further information was sought and work began in developing a suitable contrast agent.

Basic Principles of a Contrast Agent's Actions

Signal intensity and contrast between different tissues are influenced by the tissues' T1 and T2 relaxation times. The administration of a contrast agent has the effect of decreasing the relaxation times of a tissue by enhancing proton relaxation. It is not the contrast agent itself which is imaged but the effect that it has on the tissues that it concentrates in.

Contrast agents may be separated into paramagnetic and ferromagnetic agents.

Paramagnetic Agents

Paramagnetic ions possess unpaired electrons around their nuclei. These unpaired electrons generate their own strong fluctuating magnetic fields which affect the nuclear relaxation of nearby tissues.

Iron, manganese, copper, gadolinium and chromium are all examples of paramagnetic metal ions. In their free state they have been found to be too toxic for clinical use. However, linking gadolinium to a chelating agent such as diethyltriamine pentaacetic acid (Gd-DTPA; Magnevist, Schering, Berlin) lowers its toxicity and makes it clinically tolerated. Initially Gd-DTPA was the only contrast medium available, but recently other companies have completed trials using their own versions of gadolinium-based compounds using different chelates. Gd-DTPA-BMA (Omniscan, Nycomed/ Winthrop) is available in the United Kingdom; this is a non-ionic compound. Gd-HP-DO3A (Prohance, Squibb Diagnostics) and Gd-DOTA (Dotarem, Guerber, France) are two other chelates currently under evaluation.

Intravenous (i.v.) contrast medium has a distribution mechanism exactly the same as that of other iodinated X-ray contrast media. It circulates within the vascular and extracellular compartments and is rapidly excreted by glomerular filtration in the kidneys. Normally i.v. contrast medium does not cross the blood–brain barrier but concentrates in areas with no blood–brain barrier, such as the choroid plexus, pituitary stalk and nasal mucosa. In pathological conditions such as tumours, infections and demyelinating diseases, the blood–brain barrier becomes permeable to i.v. contrast medium.

Intravenous contrast medium affects both the T1 and T2 relaxation times, but it is the effect on the T1 relaxation time which is used in practice. T1-weighted images are obtained before and after intravenous administration of the i.v. contrast medium and if there is concentration of the contrast medium within the tissues being imaged (i.e. breakdown of the blood–brain barrier) then the T1-weighted images obtained show enhancement of the abnormal tissue (due to the T1 shortening). It usually takes up to 5 minutes after administration of the i.v. contrast medium to show sufficient enhancement in lesions. The effect remains for up to 45 minutes after injection, and satisfactory enhancement is still possible for up to 1 hour after injection.

The effective clinical dose has been found to be 0.2 ml per kilogram of body weight. The LD_{50} is 10 ml/kg, i.e. approximately 50% of animals die after receiving this dose. This gives a safety factor of approximately 50 times, compared with iodinated X-ray contrast media which have a safety factor of approximately 15 times.

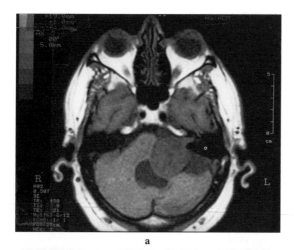

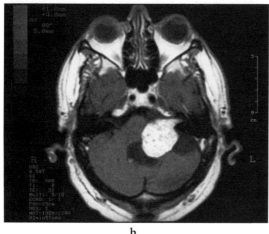

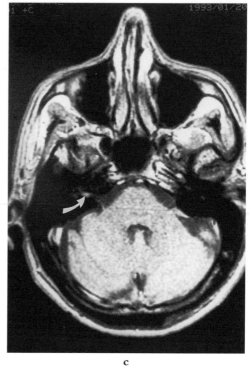

Fig. 8.1. **a** Axial SE T1-weighted image (TR 450 ms, TE 21 ms) of the posterior fossa showing a large lesion in the region of the cerebellopontine angle (CPA) which compresses the fourth ventricle and extends into the auditory canal. **b** The same sequence after administration of i.v. contrast medium shows the enhancing lesion and confirms its true extent. **c** Axial gradient echo T1-weighted image (TR 300 ms, TE 12 ms, flip angle 65°) of the posterior fossa after i.v. contrast medium shows a small intracanalicular lesion (*arrow*).

Adverse Reactions to/Tolerance of Gd-DTPA (Magnevist)

World-wide studies undertaken to determine the tolerance of Gd-DTPA have shown that it is very well tolerated. Among a total of 13 439 patients, 196 (1.45%) had adverse reactions, of which nausea and vomiting (0.42%) and local warmth/pain (0.41%) were

Table 8.1. Adverse reactions following administration of non-ionic contrast medium and Gd-DTPA

Symptoms	Non-ionic X-ray contrast media (n = 168 363)		Gd-DTPA (n = 13 439)	
Nausea/vomiting	2363	(1.4%)	57	(0.42%)
Local warmth/pain	1635	(0.97%)	55	(0.41%)
Allergy: slight reaction	1548	(0.92%)	14	(0.104%)
Allergy: mucosal	698	(0.41%)	7	(0.052%)
Flush	271	(0.16%)	8	(0.059%)

Courtesy of H.P. Niendorf, J.C. Dinger, J. Haustein et al.

the commonest. Table 8.1 shows the numbers of adverse reactions following intravenous administration of non-ionic X-ray contrast media to 168 363 patients and Gd-DTPA to 13 439 patients.

Clinical Uses of Intravenous Contrast Medium

The use of i.v. contrast medium in MRI is continually evolving and there are already too many applications to discuss here. However, we have attempted to group some of the uses of contrast in demonstrating various lesions.

Central Nervous System

The uses of i.v. contrast medium in the central nervous system include the imaging of primary and

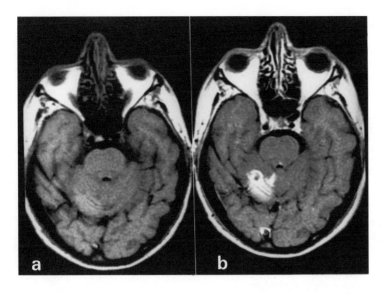

Fig. 8.2a,b. Axial SE T1-weighted images (TR 450 ms,TE 21 ms) before (**a**) and after (**b**) i.v. contrast medium showing an intracerebellar lesion which was difficult to identify on the pre-contrast image. This was found to be an abscess.

secondary tumours, infection and white matter demyelination diseases. Administration of contrast is often helpful in distinguishing tumour from oedema, and intramedullary from extramedullary lesions.

Benign tumours such as meningiomas and acoustic neuromas (Fig. 8.1) show marked enhancement with i.v. contrast medium, whilst others such as pituitary tumours, glomus jugulare tumours and epidermoid tumours may show only a small degree of enhancement.

Malignant tumours show differing amounts of enhancement depending on their degree of malignancy. Highly malignant tumours show the most enhancement in varying forms (patchy, ring, linear) and enhancement within the cystic components of tumours is not uncommon. A low-grade astrocytoma, however, will show only slight enhancement.

Infections such as abscesses (Fig. 8.2) will show ring enhancement after contrast administration. A soft tissue abscess will show ring enhancement that allows it to be distinguished from normal muscle. Paraspinal subligamentous extension of infection can be differentiated from cerebrospinal fluid and intervertebral disc (Fig. 8.3).

Demyelinating diseases such as multiple sclerosis can usually be well demonstrated on T2-weighted sequences without the administration of i.v. contrast medium. However, contrast will reveal new active plaques, owing to the recent reaction surrounding the plaque.

The administration of i.v. contrast medium to post-operative spines helps to differentiate between fibrosis and recurrent herniation (Fig. 8.4). However, this is best carried out at least 1 month following surgery when the acute post-operative changes are resolving,

making it easier to distinguish scar from disc. The enhancing epidural scar tissue can clearly show any trapped nerve roots within the scar and outlines any recurrent or residual disc fragment.

TOF angiography gives good detail of arterial vessels (as described in Chapter 7) but slow venous flow is not so well demonstrated. The T1-shortening effects of i.v. contrast medium allows the slow venous flow to be better demonstrated in TOF angiography sequences.

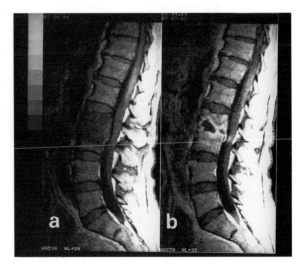

Fig. 8.3a,b. Sagittal SE T1-weighted images (TR 450 ms, TE 21 ms) before (**a**) and after (**b**) i.v. contrast medium showing loss of normal signal from the L2/3 intravertebral disc with marked enhancement of the region consistent with a diagnosis of discitis.

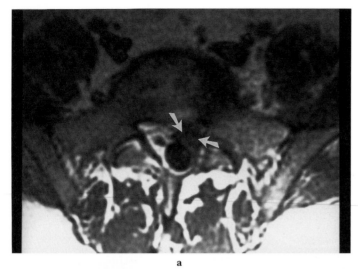

a

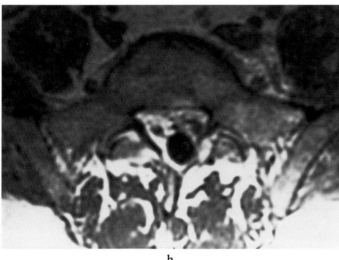

b

Fig. 8.4. **a** Axial SE T1-weighted image (TR 450 ms, TE 21 ms) of the lumbar spine in a patient who had undergone previous surgery at the level of L5/S1. There is soft tissue within the neural canal (*arrows*) with obliteration of the nerve root which could be due to either recurrent prolapsed intervertebral disc or fibrosis. **b** The same sequence after i.v. contrast medium shows enhancement of soft tissue surrounding the nerve root allowing the diagnosis of fibrosis to be made.

Head/Neck

The normal mucosa in the nasopharynx, oropharynx, sinuses and nasal cavity shows enhancement when i.v. contrast medium is administered. Highly vascular tumours such as juvenile angiofibromas will enhance markedly. Contrast enhancement in these areas is still being evaluated.

Thorax

There has been recent interest in dynamic perfusion studies of the myocardium using i.v. contrast medium, with some evidence of enhancement of the abnormal myocardium representing infarcted areas.

Although the administration of i.v. contrast medium in the evaluation of bronchogenic carcinoma is still new it has been proven that contrast makes it possible to distinguish between normal lung and tumour masses. The fact that the peak enhancement of tumour occurs slightly earlier than that of normal lung also helps to differentiate between the two. To date studies using i.v. contrast have been unable to help in the detection of metastatic lymphadenopathy.

Mammography is still the examination of choice for breast imaging, but recently dynamic MRI with i.v. contrast medium has helped to differentiate between malignant and benign lesions. Fibroadenomas show variable enhancement. Normal breast, scars and fatty lesions enhance very slightly or not at all.

Abdomen

Liver. Imaging of the liver requires a dynamic sequence as differential enhancement between tumour and normal liver occurs only in the first 2 or 3 minutes after a bolus injection of contrast medium. Delayed imaging may cause the contrast to obscure any lesions.

Kidneys. Unfortunately MRI of the renal tract is inferior to CT and is still experimental. The i.v. contrast medium increases signal within the kidneys and gives them a similar intensity to that of perirenal fat. Dynamic perfusion studies of the kidneys have recently been shown to be helpful, with characteristic enhancement showing normal excretory function. This can be very useful in evaluating the effectiveness of transplanted kidneys. It is also useful in differentiating between intrarenal and extrarenal masses.

Adrenals. Dynamic MR perfusion has shown characteristic time-dependent enhancement of benign and malignant lesions. It has been found to be superior to all other forms of imaging techniques.

Pelvis

Contrast in the bladder has a characteristic layering effect on T1-weighted images and because of its high specific gravity it concentrates in the inferior portion of the bladder (depending upon patient postion, i.e. prone or supine). The superiormost part of the bladder contains unenhanced urine and has a low signal intensity. As the contrast layers out there is an intermediate zone of high signal intensity. A third layer is sometimes seen when there is high concentration of i.v. contrast medium, and this is visualised as a marked signal loss as a consequence of superparamagnetic T2 shortening.

Intravenous contrast has not been of use in the pelvis, although dynamic perfusion studies of bladder wall tumours may prove useful.

Musculoskeletal System

Intravenous contrast medium can be used to improve the definition of bone and soft tissue tumour borders. However, T2-weighted sequences demonstrate these lesions better than T1-weighted contrast-enhanced scans and so the use of i.v. contrast medium is limited in this area.

Recent work on perfusion studies could prove helpful in lesion characterisation and the reaction to radiotherapy.

Ferromagnetic Agents

Ferromagnetism is the property of a group of atoms (unlike paramagnetism, which is the property of an individual atom) in a solid crystal. If a ferromagnetic material decreased in size to invidual particles with individual domains it will have a unique magnetic property known as "superparamagnetism".

The magnetic dipole moments of superparamagnetic compounds are much greater than those of paramagnetic compounds and so they generate local static field inhomogeneities. This causes a substantial decrease in the T2 of a tissue with little change in its T1. Superparamagnetic compounds when used with a spin echo sequence demonstrate areas of decreased signal intensity that are most obvious on T2-weighted images.

This effect is being investigated as a negative contrast agent in the gastrointestinal tract and also in the reticuloendothelial system. Ferrite (iron oxide, Fe_3O_4) is used and is targeted to the reticuloendothelial system. After intravenous administration signal loss is observed in the liver, spleen and bone marrow. It is excellent at showing tumour/liver contrast but still very much in its early days of clinical evaluation.

Research into further contrast agents is being undertaken with the hope that further targeting of agents will be possible, but it will be some time before such agents are in regular clinical use.

9 Safety and Patient Management

Safety

The statement "MRI is a totally safe imaging modality" is often made by clinicians. However, such statements are only true if certain well thought out guidelines are followed. The major safety considerations in MRI can be divided into the following groups:

1. Static magnetic field
   (a) Biological effects
   (b) Attraction effects
2. Time varying magnetic fields
3. Radiofrequency effects
4. Cryogenic effects
5. Psychological effects
6. Use of intravenous gadolinium

We will now consider each group and show their importance.

Static magnetic field

Biological Effects

A great deal of research has been done on the effects of static magnetic fields on biological tissue. Although there are currently no known effects this is by no means conclusive, as research is continuing in this area. The strength of the magnetic field plays an important role; it is stated that exposure of humans to static magnetic fields below 2.5 T is unlikely to have any adverse effects on health.

Attraction Effects

The attraction exerted by the static magnetic field on ferromagnetic objects is potentially the main safety hazard in MRI. These objects present problems both because they are strongly attracted by the high field

strengths used and because there are "fringe fields" that extend beyond the magnet bore, the extent and strength of which are determined by the type of magnet and its field strength. As described in Chapter 2, magnet shielding can be used to control the extent of the fringe field.

A field strength of 0.5 millitesla (0.5 mT; 5 gauss) is the value at which a fringe field is recognised to be safe from the risk of any attraction effects, although a fringe field of less than 0.5 mT can still affect the internal workings of pieces of equipment. Table 9.1 lists the fringe field strengths at which different devices are affected. The 0.5 mT line is recognised as the beginning of the controlled area beyond which screening of staff and patients must take place to remove any ferromagnetic objects, credit cards, etc.

Magnet shielding reduces the distances from the magnet isocentre to which fringe fields extend but a shielded magnet should never be thought of as safer than an unshielded magnet. In fact the opposite is true because there is no longer a gradual tapering of the fringe field which would give warning of the presence of a ferromagnetic object (i.e. torque of that object). Instead there is a more sudden change from a relatively low field of 3–5 mT to a field strength of several hun-

Table 9.1. The field strength at which different devices are affected

Device	Safe field strength (mT)
Videotape	3.0
Magnetic discs	
Credit cards	
Computer disc drives	1.0
X-ray tubes	
Ultrasound equipment	
Cardiac pacemaker	0.5
Multiformat camera	
X-ray image intensifiers	0.05
Gamma cameras	
CT scanners	
Linear accelerators	
Electron microscope	

dred or thousand millitesla (500–1500 mT). This means that the force exerted on the ferromagnetic object is even stronger than if there had been either no shielding or a more gradual tapering of the fringe static magnetic fields.

Since superconducting magnets are permanently energised the safety procedure employed must be followed day and night. For air core resistive magnets the fringe fields are similar to those of superconducting magnets except that they are much lower in strength in proportion to the field strength of the magnet – though this does not make them any safer once a patient is within the 0.5 mT line. Iron core resistive and permanent magnets have significantly reduced fringe fields because their iron yokes conduct the returning magnetic flux back into the imaging region and therefore, as with shielded superconducting magnets, there is a sudden increase in field strength. This means that even at the relatively lower field strengths employed, fringe field effects cannot be ignored.

Avoidance of the attraction of ferromagnetic objects to the magnet is achieved first by controlling access to the magnet room and anywhere else within the 0.5 mT line. Secondly, patients and staff must be screened for any metallic objects, implants, etc., before crossing the 0.5 mT line. A ferromagnetic metallic implant within the body may be subjected to a torque on approaching and entering the magnet, and so be potentially hazardous to the patient if dislodged from its original position. Such implants include certain types of intracranial aneurysm clips, shrapnel (especially if located near the spinal cord), intraorbital metallic foreign bodies, cochlear implants, neurostimulators, pre-1964 heart valves (Starr–Edwards) and prostheses (Table 9.2).

Cardiac Pacemakers. Patients who have undergone any cardiac surgery or who have a cardiac pacemaker *in situ* should not undergo an MRI examination. Cardiac pacemaker leads may act as antennae and result in pacing of the heart at the frequency of the applied pulse, which in turn could result in ventricular fibrillation. A pacemaker contains a relay switch called a "reed switch" the purpose of which is to switch from a synchronous to asynchronous mode of operation, and this can be activated to close when near a magnetic field. The more dependent the patient is on the uninterrupted functioning of the pacemaker the more hazardous magnetic effects become. The electrical components of the pacemaker may be damaged if subjected to RF pulses and the lithium battery itself may produce a torque effect resulting in it being dislodged.

Heart Valves. Most modern heart valves are not ferromagnetic and therefore do not present any problems.

However, valves manufactured before 1964 (Starr–Edwards) may contain ferromagnetic material and therefore be potentially dangerous.

Intraorbital Metallic Foreign Bodies. Slivers of metal within the eye may be present in patients such as welders or riveters with a history of working with metal; although superficial fragments may have been removed it is the more penetrating fragments which cause concern. These slivers may move when subjected to a magnetic field causing damage to the eye and possibly loss of vision. Radiographs of the orbit, though not quite as sensitive as CT scans, can detect intraoccular foreign bodies large enough to cause potential problems.

Intracranial Aneurysm Clips. These clips have long been recognised as a definite contraindication for an MRI examination. The torque they would experience when placed in the magnetic field could be sufficient to damage the sides of the blood vessels to which they are attached. This may result in haemorrhage, ischaemia or even death. Non-ferrous clips are now available (e.g. Sugita clips) that are safe inside the magnet. However, if there is any question about the exact type of clip a patient has then it must be assumed that it is a ferromagnetic type and the examination postponed until further information is available.

Other vascular clips may also be ferromagnetic, but it is recognised that if they have been *in situ* for 6 months or more then there will be enough fibrosis around the clip to prevent movement as the patient is advanced into the magnet. The RF as it is applied may, however, cause heating and expansion of *all* vascular clips.

It is worth noting that it is the changing magnetic fields that the patient is subjected to when moving into the bore of the magnet which cause the torque upon the foreign body, and that this torque is stronger the faster the object moves through the changing fields. A patient observed to have an unknown metallic foreign body present should be moved out of the magnet *slowly* to prevent further injury.

Projectiles. Any loose ferromagnetic objects such as hairpins, earrings, scissors, penknives, screwdrivers or keys taken into the magnet room are liable to be pulled into the magnet bore. The attractive force on such an object increases the closer it comes to the magnet. This force can cause the object to leap out of a hand or pocket before there is time to react. It is accelerated rapidly to the magnet with great force and if there were anything or anyone in the way there could be disastrous consequences. This is called the "missile effect".

Table 9.2. Classification of metallic implants for MRI

Type of implant	Deflection?	Maximum field strength tested (tesla)	Comments
Aneurysm and haemostatic clips[a]			
Drake (SS 301)	Yes	1.50	
Drake (DR 14, 24)	Yes	1.44	
Drake (DR 16)	Yes	0.15	
Drake (DR 20)	Yes	1.50	
Downs multipositional (17–7PH)	Yes	1.44	
Gastrointestinal anastomosis clip, Auto Suture SG1A (SS)	No	1.50	
Heifetz (17–7PH)	Yes	1.89	
Heifetz (Eligiloy)	No	1.89	
Hemoclip #10 (316L SS)	No	1.50	
Hemoclip (Tantalum)	No	1.50	
Housepian	Yes	0.15	
Kapp straight (SS 404)	Yes	0.15	
Kapp curved (SS 404)	Yes	1.44	
Kapp (SS 405)	Yes	1.89	
Ligaclip #6 (316L SS)	No	1.50	
Ligaclip (Tantalum)	No	1.50	
Mayfield (SS 301)	Yes	1.50	
Mayfield (SS 304)	Yes	1.89	
McFadden (SS 301)	Yes	1.50	
Olivecrona	No	1.44	
Pivot (17–7PH)	Yes	1.89	
Scoville (EN–58J)	Yes	1.89	
Stevens (50–4190 SS)	No	0.15	
Sugita (Elgiloy)	No	1.89	
Sundt–Kees (SS 301)	Yes	1.50	
Sundt–Kees multiangle (17–7PH)	Yes	1.89	
Surgiclip, Auto Suture (M–9.5)	No	1.50	
Vari-angle (17–7PH)	Yes	1.89	
Vari-angle McFadden (MP35N)	No	1.89	
Vari-angle micro (17–7PM)	Yes	0.15	
Vari-angle spring (17–7PM)	Yes	0.15	
Vari-angle (17–7PH)	Yes	1.89	
Yasargil (SS 316)	No	1.89	
Yasargil (Phynox)	No	1.89	
Heart valves[b]			
Beall	Yes	2.35	
Bjork–Shiley (convexo-concave)	No	1.50	
Bjork–Shiley (universal/spherical)	Yes	1.50	
Bjork–Shiley, model MBC	Yes	2.35	
Bjork–Shiley, model 2650	Yes	2.35	
Carpentier–Edwards, model 2650	Yes	2.35	
Carpentier–Edwards (porcine)	Yes	2.35	
Hall–Kaster, model A7700	Yes	1.50	
Hancock I (porcine)	Yes	1.50	
Hancock II (porcine)	Yes	1.50	
Hancock extracorporeal, model 242R	Yes	2.35	
Hancock extracorporeal, model M 4365–33	Yes	2.35	
Hancock Vascor, model 505	No	2.35	
Ionescu–Shiley	Yes	2.35	
Lillehi–Kaster	Yes	1.50	
Medtronic Hall	Yes	2.35	
Omnicarbon, model 3523T029	Yes	2.35	
Omniscience, model 6522	Yes	2.35	
Smeloff–Cutter	Yes	1.50	
Starr–Edwards 1260	Yes	2.35	
Starr–Edwards 2400	No	1.50	
Starr–Edwards pre 6000 (1960–1964)	Yes	1.50	Possibly contraindicated
Starr–Edwards 6520	Yes	2.35	
St. Jude	No	1.50	
St. Jude, model A 101	Yes	2.35	
St. Jude, model M 101	Yes	2.35	

(Continues)

Table 9.2. *(continued.)*

Type of implant	Deflection?	Maximum field strength tested (tesla)	Comments
Intravascular devices			
Amplatz filter	No	4.7	
Cragg Nitinol spiral filter	No	4.7	
Simon–Nitinol filter	No	1.5	
Gianturco coil (occluding spring embolus)	Yes	1.5	
Gianturco bird nest filter	Yes	1.5	High magnetic deflection
Gianturco zig-zag stent	Yes	1.5	High magnetic deflection
Greenfield vena cava filter (stainless steel)	Yes	1.5	Minimal magnetic deflection, considered safe
Greenfield vena cava filter (titanium alloy)	No	1.5	
Gunther retrievable filter	Yes	1.5	High magnetic deflection
Maas helical IVC filter	No	1.5	
Maas helical endovascular stent	No	1.5	
Mobin–Uddin filter	No	1.5	
New retrievable IVC filter	Yes	1.5	High magnetic deflection
Palmaz vascular stent	Yes	1.5	Minimal magnetic deflection
Strecker tantalum stent	No	1.5	
Orthopaedic materials/devices			
AML femoral component/bipolar hip prosthesis	No	1.5	
Charnley–Muller hip prosthesis	No	0.3	
Harris hip prosthesis	No	1.5	
Jewett nail	No	1.5	
Kirschner intermedullary rod	No	1.5	
Stainless steel plate (Zimmer)	No	1.5	
Stainless steel screw (Zimmer)	No	1.5	
Stainless steel mesh	No	1.5	
Stainless steel wire	No	1.5	
Dental materials			
Dental amalgam	No	1.44	
Brace band	No	1.50	
Brace wire	Yes	1.50	Probably safe for MRI
Gutta percha points	No	1.50	
Indian head real silver points	No	1.50	
Temporary crown	No	1.50	
Permanent crown amalgam	No	1.50	
Prosthetic ear implants			
Cody tack	No	0.6	
Cochlear implant (3M/House)	Yes	0.6	Contraindicated
Cochlear implant (3M/Vienna)	Yes	0.6	Contraindicated
House-type incus prosthesis	No	0.6	
McGee stainless steel piston	No	0.6	
Reuter drain tube	No	0.6	
Richards–McGee piston	No	1.5	
Richards–Schuknecht Teflon wire	No	1.5	
Richards plasti-pore with Armstrong-style platinum ribbon	No	1.5	
Richards trapeze platinum ribbon	No	1.5	
Richards House-type wire loop	No	1.5	
Xomed stapes prosthesis, Robinson-style	No	1.5	
Schuknecht gel foam and wire prosthesis, Armstrong-style	No	1.5	
Penile implants			
AMS malleable 600	No	1.5	
AMS 700 CX	No	1.5	
Flexi-flate (Surgitek)	No	1.5	
Flexi-rod (standard) (Surgitek)	No	1.5	
Flexi-rod II (firm) (Surgitek)	No	1.5	
Jonas (Dacomed)	No	1.5	
Mentor flexible	No	1.5	
Mentor inflatable	No	1.5	
Omniphase (Dacomed)	Yes	1.5	

(Continues)

Table 9.2. *(continued.)*

Type of implant	Deflection?	Maximum field strength tested (tesla)	Comments
Miscellaneous			
AMS 800, artificial sphincter	No	1.50BBs	Yes 1.50
Bullet (steel tip)	Yes	1.50	
Cerebral ventricular shunt tube connector, Accu-Flow, straight (Codman and Shurtleff)	No	1.50	
Cerebral ventricular shunt tube connector, Accu-Flow, right angle (Codman and Shurtleff)	No	1.50	
Cerebral ventricular shunt tube connector, Accu-Flow, T-connector (Codman and Shurtleff)	No	1.50	
Cerebral ventricular shunt tube connector (type unknown)	Yes	0.15	
Diaphragm (all flex)	Yes	1.50	Probably safe for MRI
Diaphragm (Ortho)	Yes	1.50	Probably safe for MRI
Diaphragm (Koroflex)	Yes	1.50	Probably safe for MRI
Diaphragm (titanium)	No	1.44	
Forceps (titanium)	No	1.44	
Hakim valve and pump	No	1.44	
Infusaid implantable chemotherapy pump	No	1.50	Safe for MRI
Intraocular lens implant, iridocapsular lens, plantinum–iridium loop (Binkhorst)	No	1.00	
Intraocular lens implant, iridocapsular lens, titanium loop (Binkhorst)	No	1.00	
Intraocular lens implant, platinum clip lens (Worst)	No	1.00	
IUD copper T	No	1.50	
IUD copper 7	No	1.50	
Tantalum powder	No	1.44	
Thermodilution catheter (Swan-Ganz VIP, 5 Fr, 7Fr)	No	1.50	May still be unsafe owing to possibility of induced current
Vitallium implant	No	1.50	

Courtesy of Edelman & Hesselink (1990).

Magnetic properties of implants. Most implants that demonstrate no deflection in a magnetic field are safe for MRI. However, some implants (e.g. pacemakers, cochlear implants, neurostimulators) are still contraindicated because the magnetic field may produce electronic malfunction. Note that the presence of deflection does not necessarily represent a contraindication to MRI, particularly if such devices are firmly fixed in position (e.g. by surgical means or fibrosis). However, clinical judgment should be exercised before imaging such implants. In addition, note that absence of deflection at a lower field strength does not preclude deflection at a higher field strength.

[a] Note that certain nominally non-ferromagnetic clips may produce substantial image artifacts due to local distortion of the RF field or to mild ferromagnetism induced by bending of the clips during placement.

[b] Magnetic deflection forces probably not significant compared with mechanical stresses in vivo, with the possible exception of older Starr–Edwards models in patients with valvular dehiscence.

Large ferromagnetic objects such as trolleys, wheelchairs, oxygen cylinders and anaesthetic machines have been known to be accidentally pulled into the magnet. There are other objects such as watches and bleeps which should not be taken into the magnet room as they can be permanently damaged. Domestic staff should be fully aware of the dangers and all cleaning equipment must be non-magnetic.

The correct precautions must be taken to ensure that such accidents do not occur. This includes the use of non-magnetic equipment for wheelchairs, trolleys, anaesthetic machines, etc. Metal detectors are used at some sites to check patients and staff, but they are not sensitive enough to detect small ferromagnetic objects and so cannot be relied upon totally.

Time Varying Magnetic Fields

The gradient coils in the MR system which are used to spatially locate the signal are switched on and off rapidly during a pulse sequence. The strength of these gradient fields is very small compared with that of the main magnetic field (typically 1–10 mT/m), but their rate of change in the magnetic field (dB) per unit time (dt) causes induced currents (according to Faraday's law) and is a potential safety hazard. The gradient switching is done for periods of 1 ms or less which results in field variations of 5.0–2.5 T/s.

The biological effects of these induced currents are both a result of the power they deposit and a direct result of the currents themselves. If the induced currents are large enough they may cause stimulation of both nerve and muscle cells. This can result in ventricular fibrillation, visual field sensations (magnetophosphenes), epilepsy and bone healing. Individuals will vary in their sensitivity to induced currents, especially if they are receiving neuroactive medication or have a neurological disorder. Further research is being carried out in this area.

A clear document should be supplied from the manufacturer indicating the maximum operating values of the gradients (dB/dt) that the equipment will allow under normal conditions and also maximum values if a fault occurs. The manufacturer should also guarantee that the recommended levels will not be exceeded unless deliberately overridden by the operator. The threshold currents required to produce nerve stimulation, ventricular, fibrillation, etc., far exceed those used in present MR systems. Echoplanar imaging involves the use of much more rapid changes in the gradient fields and recent studies have shown peripheral muscle stimulation in humans at a threshold of 60 T/s.

Acoustic Levels

Another factor which needs to be taken into account is the noise level. There is characteristic noise produced within the MR system during data acquisition. This is caused by the switching on and off of the gradients, which results in their vibration against the cryostat with an associated banging noise. The amplitude of this noise can vary depending on the design of the magnet, the pulse sequence chosen, pulse sequence timing and the amount of current passing through the coils (which is operator controlled depending upon field of view, slice thickness and pulse sequence). The acceptable noise level from a clinical MR system is between 65 and 95 decibels (db). There have, however, been reports of temporary and permanent hearing loss as a result of an MRI examination. Ear plugs should be readily available to offer patients some protection. Phase cancellation techniques are being developed in which the sound emitted from the gradients is analysed and a noise of the same amplitude and frequency but with an opposite phase is generated to cancel it out.

Noise is also produced by the shield cooler unit, but this is considerably lower in amplitude and not considered to be clinically significant.

Radiofrequency Effects

RF is used to excite the hydrogen protons in the body tissues during MRI. The energy absorbed by the pro-

tons is dissipated as heat, but it is such a small amount that it is of no clinical concern. The RF, being an oscillating electrical and magnetic field, induces electrical currents within the tissues of the patient. The majority of the RF is transformed into heat within these tissues and it is the thermal biological effects which are mainly of relevance to MRI.

If heating occurs within human tissues then the body's thermoregulatory devices sense it and there is a localised dilation of blood vessels, resulting in increased blood flow with the removal of excess heat from the body, mainly at the skin surface. The lens of the eye is a notable exception: being completely avascular it is unable to lose heat at the same rate as other tissues.

The rise in temperature of the tissue depends upon the rate of absorption of the RF energy and its rate of dissipation. Specific absorption rates (SAR) of 0.4 watts per kilogram (W/kg) for the whole body and 8.0 W/kg for any 1 g of tissue are acceptable. For the head a SAR of 3.2 W/kg or less is below the critical level. The rise in body temperature caused by RF power is more critical in some areas than others. The testes are particularly sensitive to temperature changes, laboratory investigations having demonstrated detrimental temperature-related effects on testicular function (cessation of spermatogenesis, impairment of sperm mobility and degeneration of seminiferous tubules). However, the temperature changes encountered in clinical MRI are too small to impair spermatogenesis. In the lens, laboratory tests have demonstrated cataract formation in animals, but with the RF power encountered in clinical MRI the temperature rises are well within the threshold limits.

To prevent temperature damage to tissues the recommended safe temperature levels are as follows:

Maximum whole body (core) temperature rise should be less than 1 °C.

Localised heating should be no greater than 38 °C in the head, 39 °C in the trunk and 40 °C in the extremities.

The increase in tissue temperature from the RF field is a result of a series of variable factors including: duration of exposure, humidity, air flow around the patient in the magnet, the rate at which energy is deposited and the background temperature.

RF Burns

There have been several reports of first, second and third degree burns resulting from a clinical MRI examination and therefore it is necessary to take precautionary measures routinely. Obvious exposed wires or conductors should never touch any part of the patient and no induced current loops should be formed that in any way directly involve any part of the patient e.g. ECG monitoring or gating leads and the patient's skin. Unconnected imaging coils should not be left within the magnet during imaging as these can be a source of conduction. Insulating material should be placed between the wires exiting from the magnet system and the patient so that there is no direct contact at any time.

Cryogenic Effects

Liquid helium and, in older magnets, liquid nitrogen are used to maintain the required temperatures of the superconducting magnet coils. Although improvement in cryostat design has eliminated the use of liquid nitrogen it is still necessary to be aware of the effects of any inadvertent leak of either of these cryogens.

Magnets Using Helium Only

Liquid helium will achieve a gaseous state at approximately -268.92 °C (4.2 K). If for any reason the temperature of the cryostat rises then there will be a sudden rapid "boil off" of the helium. The marked increase in volume associated with the change to the gaseous state would increase the pressure within the cryostat and result in a pressure-sensitive valve blowing, allowing the excess gas to be vented out of the building and into the atmosphere. If the valve fails to work or a seal is broken then the gas could leak into the magnet room. The helium, which is considerably lighter than air, would rise into the room in a characteristic cloud (being so cold). If sufficient helium escapes into the magnet room then frost bite could occur, followed by asphyxiation if exposure was for a long period.

Magnets Using Liquid Nitrogen and Helium

Liquid nitrogen achieves a gaseous state at -196 °C (77.3 K). Nitrogen has approximately the same density as air and if allowed to escape into the magnet room is more likely than helium to settle at floor level. Frost bite is one possible danger from such an event. Pure nitrogen is extremely hazardous and unconsciousness would result after 5–10 seconds of exposure, death occurring within a few minutes.

It is imperative that if a leak of either helium or nitrogen occurs all patients and staff evacuate the area as soon as possible and do not return until the leak has been found and repaired.

To help in the detection of leaks an oxygen monitor which measures the percentage of oxygen in the air should always be in position at head height in the magnet room. The monitor should have an audible alarm which sounds if the oxygen percentage saturation falls below a pre-set level. In association with this an automatic link to a ventilation system which would start extracting air if the alarm sounded is something to be considered when planning an MRI site. Any leakage of cryogens within the magnet room would result in a secondary increase in pressure within the room to such a degree that there may be some difficulty opening the door. If this problem is encountered while there is a patient in the scanner some means of equalising the pressure must be found, such as breaking the observation window. This situation may be avoided altogether if the site incorporates an emergency extraction system.

The helium and nitrogen levels are monitored by meters which give radiographers and physicists the opportunity to make daily checks. From these the daily, weekly and monthly consumption of the cryogens can be determined. This means that any increase in consumption can be identified and brought to the attention of the service personnel and investigated in case of a leak. The cryogens in the cryostat need to be refilled periodically; this procedure must be carried out by suitably qualified and equipped personnel who follow strict guidelines in order to avoid spillage.

Quenches

A quenching facility is provided to allow an emergency shutdown of the magnetic field. A switch is situated in the magnet room which, when activated, causes the magnetic field to cease abruptly. This is achieved by applying heat to a superconducting switch which causes resistance within the magnet windings; further heating of these windings then occurs very rapidly. The liquid helium will evaporate, a process usually accompanied by a loud bang and the evolution of large quantities of cold gas which escapes via a vent into the atmosphere.

Psychological Effects

The major psychological effect experienced by patients undergoing an MRI examination is claustrophobia with associated panic attacks. It is difficult to put an exact figure on the number of patients affected owing to the varying degrees of claustrophobia, from a mild "initial panic but managed to go through with it" to a severe "help get me out!" situation. The number of patients who have refused to have their examination at our MRI unit is a fraction of 1% of the total patients scanned.

The feeling of claustrophobia can result from several factors: being left alone, being enclosed, fear of the unknown, the noise associated with the MRI system, and the overall scan time. Most of these problems can be alleviated by having a well-planned patient preparation and management procedure from the moment that the patient's appointment is made. This procedure should include the following:

1. An accurate patient information leaflet sent out with the appointment that describes the machines, its mode of operation, contraindications and also what is expected of the patient during the scan. Photographs of the scanner should be included in this leaflet to give the patient an idea of what to expect.

2. A pre-appointment visit to the MRI unit if required for patients who fear they may be claustrophobic or for children whose parents do not know whether the child will be able to cooperate.

3. A time when the patient arrives for his or her appointment during which the radiographer should try to put the patient at ease and answer any queries. If the patient is anxious or requests it, a relative or friend should be allowed to stay in the room with them during the examination.

4. The use of mirrors mounted inside the scanner to allow the patient to see out of the scanner.

5. The maintenance of verbal or, if necessary, physical contact with the patient throughout the examination.

6. Possible use of a blindfold to prevent the patient from seeing into the magnet.

7. Possible use of the prone position for the patient so that he or she can see out of the magnet.

8. Music to help to relax the patient.

9. Availability of ear-plugs to help reduce the noise.

The comparatively small cost involved in setting up a suitable safe system is a worthwhile investment.

Continuing improvements in magnet design (larger diameters, shorter bores) may help reduce claustrophobia.

Use of Intravenous Gadolinium

Magnevist (Schering Health Care Ltd) and Omniscan (Nycomed UK) are currently the only two contrast agents licensed in the United Kingdom. They both have a very high safety factor and patient tolerance level compared with iodinated contrast media.

Among the reactions related to the administration of Gd-DTPA are headache, nausea, vomiting, hives and a local burning sensation. In cases where the contrast has been extravasated there may be local reactions. However, there have been cases reported where erythema, swelling and pain at the site of injection had a delayed onset of 1–4 days. There have been rare reports of anaphylactoid reactions and also a very small number of deaths in which the relationship of the drug, the patient's condition and the cause of death are still being investigated. To date there are not enough data available to assess the safety of Gd-DTPA in pregnant women but gadolinium has been known to cross the placenta and appear in the fetal bladder.

The recommended dose for head and spinal imaging is 0.1 mmol/kg body weight, which is the equivalent of 0.2 ml/kg. Recently higher concentrations have been licensed for use; it is claimed that these have greater sensitivity in lesion detection. The lethal dose is 10 ml/kg body weight.

Emergency Procedures

Having discussed the various safety concerns associated with the MRI scanner we should now consider how the local hospital environment interacts with the MRI unit. Local rules should be drawn up to cater for the emergency situations of cardiac arrest in the patient and fire.

Cardiac Arrest

In the event of a patient suffering a cardiac arrest in the scanner resuscitation, i.e. cardiac massage and maintaining an airway, can begin in the magnet room but the patient should be removed from the scanner and moved to an area outside the 0.5 mT line where resuscitation can continue by a qualified team. The risk of ferrous resuscitation equipment in the magnet room is too great and should *never* be considered.

Fire

In the event of a fire the department should be evacuated of all patients and staff after the alarm has been raised. If at all possible any electrical equipment and mains isolators should be switched off. If the fire is situated in the magnet room or if access to the magnet room is required by the emergency services then the magnet should be quenched or turned off prior to admittance. Permanent magnet systems cannot be switched off but their fringe fields are low compared with those of other magnet systems. Clear warnings should be placed around the fringe field to indicate its presence. Resistive and superconducting magnets should also have warning notices to indicate their fringe fields as in certain circumstances the magnet may not need to be switched off.

Smoke detectors placed around the rooms may help to prevent a serious fire.

It may be practicable to instal a Halon fire extinguisher system which can be manually activated in the event of a fire. This may eliminate the need to quench the magnet and also reduce other damage to the magnet and the department. All patients and staff must have been evacuated from the area before the Halon gas system is activated.

Informing fire officers and chiefs of the nature of the equipment and the potential risks involved is critical. This may prevent any misunderstanding occurring in the event of a fire.

Patient Management

We have already mentioned the need for good patient management when considering the psychological effects of the MRI examination. It is worthwhile considering this in greater detail.

The patient is the most important part of the MRI examination. Gaining the patient's cooperation and confidence is a skill that often goes unappreciated: the equipment may be the most modern available but its benefits cannot be realised without the complete cooperation of the patient.

Clinical MRI scanners are built to provide a service for clinicians which in turn provides information and benefits for the patients under their care. It is therefore of paramount importance that the service is geared to provide this information as efficiently as possible.

The process begins when the clinician brings the request card to the department. This request card should contain the relevant personal patient information, as with any X-ray request card. Also included are a number of questions regarding any possible contraindications to the examination, such as pacemakers, pregnancy, surgical clips and prostheses. The clinician should discuss the request with the radiologist, who should then make recommendations as to any particular protocols required and acknowledge this on the card, as well as the urgency of the examination.

The next step is to make the patient an appointment, bearing in mind the urgency of the request, the distance the patient has to travel, whether the patient will be coming by ambulance and the age of the patient. A patient information leaflet should be sent to the patient together with the appointment date. It is good practice to ask the patient to confirm the

Table 9.3. Patient checklist

Name of patient:
Weight:
Address:
Date of birth:

Have you ever had any previous X-ray examinations in this hospital?   Yes/No
Please give dates:

Do you have a cardiac pacemaker/heart valve replacement?   Yes/No

Do you have a cochlear implant?   Yes/No

Have you ever had any operations on your head or spine?   Yes/No
Please give approximate dates:

Have you ever had any operations which might involve the use of any metallic pins/plates/clips or screws?   Yes/No

Have you ever had an injury which involved metal fragments/filings in relation to your eyes/face or spine?   Yes/No
Please give dates and action taken:

Female patients:
Is there any possibility that you might be pregnant?   Yes/No
Number of weeks:

Check completed by:
Date:

appointment 2 days beforehand; the patient can also ring the department before leaving home to check that the scanner is working, especially if they have any distance to travel.

On arriving in the department the patient will be asked to book in at the reception desk, where the receptionist will check their particulars and direct them to the MRI waiting area. It is now the turn of the radiographer to meet the patient and, although this has already been done at reception, to check their particulars to ensure it is the correct patient. Now is the time to try to put the patient at ease and to answer any questions they may have, as well as discussing the procedure with them and what they may expect. As previously mentioned claustrophobia is the main problem encountered; a few extra words of encouragement at this stage may help later. Each patient must be thoroughly checked to ensure they are suitable for undergoing an MRI scan and a precise list of questions (checklist) should be answered. Table 9.3 gives examples of questions to be considered in compiling a checklist. If the answer to any of the questions is "Yes" then further details should be obtained and the MRI examination delayed until the query is discussed with a radiologist.

The patient is asked to remove any metallic objects from their person; these should be secured in a locker. If necessary the patient is asked to change into a gown or a suitable item of clothing they may have brought with them. Bras or dentures must be removed; even a small metallic clip on a bra can cause degradation of the images. Eye make-up can sometimes contain ferromagnetic iron and therefore produce artifacts as well as the possibility of eye irritation. Patients can be asked in the patient information leaflet not to wear eye make-up, or it may be removed if necessary on arrival at the unit.

The patient is now ready. After a final check that nothing metallic has been carried in with them, they can enter the magnet room. At this point the patient may feel like running away and so encouragement and reassurance is still essential. It is important to take as much time as the patient needs when positioning them on the table; if music is requested they can be given headphones. Keep talking to them as they are moved into the magnet bore; the patient must realise that if they call out you will be able to hear them. An emergency button is available which the patient can hold and press for assistance.

When the scanning procedure has been completed the patient is likely to become anxious about the results. It is important to indicate to the patient how they obtain their results and how long they may expect to wait.

It is obviously important that the patient's details are correctly labelled on the films and it should be indicated whether contrast medium has been administered. Also the sequences used and the scanning parameters should be recorded. A record of the patient and the examination should be logged and stored for archival permanence on a suitable medium such as optical disc or magnetic tape.

After the film has been processed and the details checked against the card once again, the films are displayed for the radiologist to report on. The checking should not stop here; the radiologist is also responsible for ensuring that the card and films are correct for that patient. Once the results have been reported a copy of the report should be sent out immediately to the clinician so that the patient does not have to wait unnecessarily. The films and report should be filed until required again.

As mentioned in Chapter 5 it is important to monitor the hard copies as well as the whole imaging system in order to produce high-quality diagnostic images. Of equal importance is the monitoring of the rest of the service provided. Patient questionnaires can be valuable in assessing how well the service is being run and may also highlight any deficiencies.

Regular staff meetings are essential to keep staff up to date and to allow them to air any queries. It can also be useful to obtain feedback from clinicians as to the efficiency of the service provided.

Many of the considerations in planning new installations for CT scanning or any other imaging modality apply also to planning an MRI suite. However, because of the nature of its operation there are a number of other factors which need to be taken into consideration in site planning for MRI.

Site planning of MRI suites is undertaken by equipment manufacturers. Modern computer-aided design (CAD) software allows both manufacturer and purchaser to consider various options in making the best use of the space available. Performance, cost and space requirements are important when investing in an MRI scanner; cost and space may be the key factors in any compromise required. Efficiency in MRI is determined by image quality, patient throughput and operating cost. An investment in an MRI scanner should be protected by the manufacturers against obsolescence, i.e. upgrades in an evolving technology should be available.

This chapter aims to help the radiographer and radiologist understand the various factors which have to be considered. It will also outline the major concerns in site planning and the issues behind them. These will be considered under the following headings:

1. Location
2. The magnet
3. The fringe field
4. RF shielding
5. Equipment
6. Patient and staff requirements

Location

Not so long ago MRI scanners had to be sited in a "green area" away from all other equipment. However, as a result of improvements in magnet design and the variety of field strengths available there are probably few locations which cannot now be adapted to house an MRI system of some description.

The Magnet

The question most often asked with regard to MRI magnets is "Which field strength should I choose?" This is difficult to answer as no single field strength can offer all possible benefits or fit all the needs of every department. The most suitable type of magnet and the field strength will depend upon the requirements of the scanner (i.e. whether it is for clinical use, research, spectroscopy or mobile imaging); the siting of the magnet will in turn depend upon the type and strength of magnet chosen.

Image quality is a very important consideration and this is determined by the signal-to-noise ratio (SNR), contrast resolution and the absence of artifacts. It might be though that, because the SNR increases with field strength, the higher the field strength then the better the image quality. There are, however, other issues which affect image quality namely chemical shift artifacts, RF power deposition, T1 relaxation times, inhomogeneities of the main field and safety. These all increase proportionally with field strength and have a detrimental effect on the images. (Resolution in spectroscopy, however, increases with field strength, resulting in improved separation between the individual lines of a spectrum.)

To produce a good-quality image the magnetic field needs to be uniform in the bore of the magnet. To achieve this the magnet is adjusted to compensate for ferrous materials, such as steel joists, in the vicinity of the scanner which may affect its performance by generating stray magnetic fields.

Types of Magnet

Superconducting Magnets

The magnets most commonly employed are superconducting magnets. Field strengths from 0.35 T to 2 T are commercially available, with one research magnet of 4 T in use. The merits of superconducting magnets have been discussed in Chapter 2; from the point of view of site planning, they present a number of problems which have to be allowed for.

First, cryogens are required within the magnet and refilling the cryostat with cryogens must be undertaken periodically. Cryogens are supplied in large insulated non-magnetic dewars. Access to the magnet room is required for these dewars, as is a storage site for them. Refrigeration units can be used instead of employing liquid nitrogen to maintain the helium at the required temperature. Reliquefaction units are available which re-liquefy the evaporated helium and return it to the helium reservoir. This removes the need for the periodic cryogen fills but is an expensive undertaking.

We mentioned in Chapter 9 the requirement for quenching a superconductive magnet in an emergency. Obviously when planning a site such requirements as an escape vent into the atmosphere must be allowed for. Possible asphyxia from the cryogens in the event of a leak should be anticipated in the site planning, i.e. oxygen sensors and air extraction systems need to be installed.

Typically superconducting magnets weigh anything from 6 to 15 tonnes. With the addition of full shielding this can increase to 40 tonnes on average, and at these weights structural alterations have to be considered. Unshielded magnets will probably not require any structural reinforcement to an existing building. The size and weight of a superconducting magnet means that it will probably have to be sited with the use of a crane and therefore access to the building must be available. Also, in the event of a magnet fault or replacement allowance must be made in the architecture of the building for the magnet's removal.

The fringe field of a superconducting magnet, which is generated in three dimensions outside the magnet bore, is an important factor when considering site design. These fringe fields are much larger than with resistive or permanent magnets due to the higher field strengths obtained (see below).

Resistive Magnets

The field strengths of resistive magnets vary according to their design but are usually from 0.01 T up to 0.4 T. Water cooling systems are used in resistive magnets to aid in cooling the magnet windings, and power consumption in these magnets is very high (100 kW). Resistive magnets weigh about 4 tonnes and so do not require floor reinforcement. These magnets can be switched off when not in use.

Permanent Magnets

Permanent magnets operate at field strengths as high as

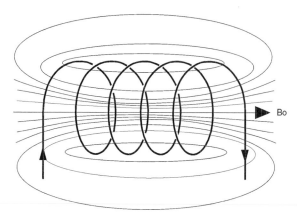

Fig. 10.1.   The magnetic lines of force around a solenoid coil.

0.3 T. This type of magnet can be transported in pieces and assembled on site. However, they weigh up to 100 tonnes and therefore need special reinforcement, which can be expensive. No current is required to maintain the magnetic field but power is needed for other parts of the system. Cooling devices are not necessary as there is no heat production. This type of magnet is relatively cheap to run.

The Fringe Field

Fringe fields were discussed in detail in Chapter 9. We will now compare the fringe fields in superconducting, resistive and permanent magnet systems.

Fringe Fields in Different Types of Magnet

Superconducting Magnets

The fringe fields produced by superconducting magnets present more of a problem than those associated with resistive or permanent magnets due to the higher field strengths of the systems and the solenoid design of the magnet. Fig. 10.1 shows the magnetic lines of force around a solenoid coil – the same design that a superconducting magnet follows.

Since fringe fields are three-dimensional careful consideration is needed when siting the magnet, as these fields can interfere with equipment above, below or around the magnet. In other words care must be taken when choosing the site to protect the environment from the fringe fields as well as to protect the magnet itself from the environment.

Resistive Magnets

The fringe fields of air core resistive magnets are very similar to those of a superconducting magnet. However, because they generate much weaker magnetic fields they affect a much smaller volume.

Iron core and permanent resistive magnets have a minimal fringe field compared with resistive air core and superconducting magnets. The reason for this is that instead of the magnetic lines of force spreading outwards they are conducted back into the magnet by its design. Fig. 10.2 shows the magnetic lines of force of a permanent magnet and demonstrates the minimal fringe field produced.

Ferromagnetic Objects

The performance of the magnet can be affected by ferromagnetic objects that are either static or moving. Static ferromagnetic objects include reinforced concrete and iron joists or girders, and these affect the magnetic lines of force and consequently the homogeneity of the magnet causing degradation of the images. Specialised shimming procedures can help to compensate for some of these objects. Complex computer programs can be used by equipment manufacturers to assess the distortion of the fringe field at the proposed site and will help to determine whether these distortions can be compensated for by shimming.

Moving ferromagnetic objects such as cars, lorries and lifts cannot be compensated for by shimming and so must be kept at a predetermined distance to ensure homogeneity of the magnet.

Devices Affected by Fringe Fields

The fringe field can affect the workings of other nearby equipment including vital medical devices (such as patient monitoring equipment and respirators), CT scanners, image intensifiers and colour television monitors, and can lead to erasure of information stored on magnetic tapes or floppy disks. Attention must be given also to implanted devices such as cardiac pacemakers and insulin pumps. The distances from the magnet at which such equipment starts to be affected should be assessed by the manufacturers before installation.

Shielding

Magnet shielding will help to confine the fringe fields to a smaller volume but can be costly. There are several types of shielding available:

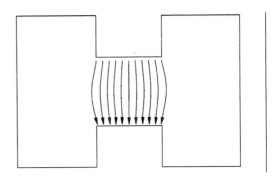

Fig. 10.2. The magnetic lines of force of a permanent magnet.

1. *Active shielding*. This can reduce the fringe fields by up to 95% and allows magnets to be sited in smaller areas.
2. *Self shielding*. Unfortunately this can weigh as much as 21 tonnes and therefore increases the need for floor reinforcement. However, it will reduce the fringe fields by about 50%.
3. *Room shielding*. This is expensive and because of the added weight also requires structural alterations and reinforcement.
4. *Partial shielding*. When only a limited area of the environment is affected by the fringe field, an appropriately positioned steel plate can "pull in" that part of the field.

Further details on magnet shielding are given in Chapter 2.

RF Shielding

When planning an MRI site not only the magnetic fringe fields have to be considered but also the RF shield. RF shielding should be considered from two different aspects: (1) protection of the environment from the RF produced by the scanner and (2) protection of the scanner from the RF present in the atmosphere from such sources as TV transmitters, commercial radio stations and emergency service radios.

Protection is provided by blocking the RF before it reaches the atmosphere or imager. This is usually achieved by containing the scanning room in an RF-shielded enclosure consisting of a continuous metal sheet (usually copper) which is grounded (earthed) at one point. The copper need be only a very thin foil to provide an adequate barrier. At certain places the enclosure is modified to allow entry of patients and (separately) the entry of electrical wires, anaesthetic gases, etc. There are alternative shielding methods which only partially surround the magnet and so have the advantage of being considerably cheaper but the disadvantage of preventing access to the back of the magnet as they cover one end.

Prior to installation an RF survey should be undertaken of the proposed site to indicate the level of RF interference and thus the level of shielding required. Typically attenuation of 90–1110 decibels is sufficient (equivalent to attenuation of interfering signals by a factor of approximately 100 000).

Engineering firms manufacture prefabricated RF shielded rooms with which to line the walls of the scanning room. The joins are usually soldered to form a continuous electrical connection. The doors to the scanning room must be specially constructed with a sheet of copper foil within them. In order to make the electrical connection between the door and the adjacent walls and floor, copper spring-loaded "fingers" line the edges of the door and maintain a continuous electrical contact when the door is closed. Windows are necessary to allow visual monitoring of the patient in the scanner. RF shielding is provided by two finely perforated sheets of copper (painted matt black) placed between two sheets of window glass.

Access of any electrical or ducting devices must be achieved via a special "RF penetration panel". If a hole were simply drilled in the RF shield for an electrical wire to pass through then the wire would act as an antenna picking up RF interference from outside the shielded room and transmitting it along its length, with potentially disastrous consequences. Instead all connections pass through an RF penetration panel into the RF shielded room. The panel also allows further access at a later date if required, rather than having to break the RF shield at another point.

Access to the magnet room for pipes, ventilation and heating ducts is achieved with lengths of copper tubing known as "wave guides" which are soldered to the RF penetration panel. For this tubing to be effective its length must be five or six times its diameter. The wave guides form an effective barrier as long as their contents are not electrically conducting. Modifications of this design, in which much shorter and smaller-diameter tubes running parallel to each other still form an effective barrier, are used to allow ventilation ducts to penetrate the shielding. The vent/duct for escaping cryogens is also a modified wave guide.

Electrical penetrations of the RF shield can be achieved by using a special "low pass line filter". This device allows direct current and low-frequency alternating current to pass through it whilst acting as a bar-

rier to the higher frequencies which would interfere with the MR signal. Low pass filters are available for a variety of different voltages and currents. They are mounted on the RF penetration panel so that the filtered wires pass directly from the filter into the RF shielded room. An alternative to low pass filters is to convert the electrical signal to a fibre-optic signal. This can penetrate the RF shield via a fibre-optic cable within a wave guide and be converted back to an electrical signal inside the RF shielded room.

There are alternative methods of RF shielding. Two manufacturers provide a retractable RF shield which covers half the length of the patient table (magnet end). The cover is electrically connected to the magnet housing and there is an RF shield beneath the table too. The opposite end of the magnet has an RF shield over the bore. This system operates on the same principle as the RF wave guides but, due to the fact that the patient conducts some RF interference, is not as effective as an RF shielded room. It is, however, much cheaper. The manufacturers feel that the RF shielding provided by such a system is sufficient for imaging purposes, quoting attenuation factors of 80 decibels.

Another method recently developed consists of a smaller RF shielded room containing the patient table. The magnet itself is located adjacent to the RF shielded room, with the magnet housing electrically connected to the room. The opposite end of the magnet has RF shielding over the bore. This type of RF shielding is advantageous as it means that the RF shielded room no longer needs to be very high to allow access for cryogen refills. It also has the advantage of a lower financial outlay.

Equipment manufacturers employ engineering firms with experience of providing RF shielded rooms to carry out strenuous testing of the completed shielding. This ensures that the RF shielding is providing sufficient attenuation and allows any suspect areas to be located and repaired.

Equipment

Any item required in the magnet room needs to be non-magnetic. Some materials become strongly magnetised when placed in a magnetic field (e.g. iron, nickel, cobalt, ferrites); the amount of nickel in an alloy will determine its ferromagnetism. Some stainless steel is non-magnetic but not all, depending upon the proportion of chromium and nickel present.

Aluminium, on the other hand, is completely non-magnetic.

Care must be taken to choose suitable magnet-safe equipment. All wheelchairs, trolleys and drip stands must be made of a non-magnetic material as must all floor cleaning equipment, ladders and tools. No electric floor polishers or cleaners should be allowed in the magnet room and no aerosol cans.

Resuscitation equipment cannot be used in the magnet room as ECG machines and defibrillators are magnetic. It is also not possible to intubate a patient in the magnet room as the magnetic effect on the batteries of the laryngoscope may prevent it from operating correctly. There would be no time to check the resuscitation team for metallic objects and so in the event of an emergency it is best to get the patient out of the scanner onto a non-magnetic trolley and take them to a safe area.

Patient and Staff Requirements

Patient Requirements

The scanning room should be as bright and airy as possible and the decor tasteful. Pictures and mobiles may help to make the room look more friendly and music can be available to the patient to help them to relax whilst in the scanner. A good intercom system so that patient and staff can communicate with each other and a hand-held emergency button which the patient can press for assistance may help to reassure the patient.

The floor should be non-slip and there should be adequate space around the scanning table to manoeuvre the non-magnetic trolley. Adequate cupboard space should be available to house the surface coils, pads, test objects, clean linen, etc.

There should be a well-decorated patient waiting room with reading material and facilities for making hot drinks in case the patient has had a long journey or is kept waiting unavoidably. A good-sized patient changing area with toilet facilities suitable for the disabled and security lockers for patients' belongings are required. Patients may bring their own clothing to change into, but if they do not then clean gowns, dressing gowns and plastic shoes should be at hand.

If space allows, a recovery room for anaesthetised or poorly patients is advantageous as this can avoid the loss of scanning time that results if the patient has to be anaesthetised in the control room.

Staff Requirements

The requirements for staff are as follows:

1. Changing area and toilets.
2. Security lockers for personal belongings.
3. Light, well-ventilated work areas.
4. Easy access to patients in the scanning room and waiting room.
5. Suitable well-marked fire exits/doors.
6. Sink with hot and cold running water.
7. Refrigerator for drugs.
8. Telephone.
9. Closed circuit television system for patient monitoring and a patient viewing window.
10. Storage cupboards, bench space, bookshelves, etc.
11. Adjustable-height chairs.
12. Viewing boxes positioned away from monitors (to prevent unwanted reflections).

Anaesthesia in MRI

Anaesthesia in MRI presents several problems which are not encountered in other departments. Even the simplest task of monitoring a patient can prove difficult because of RF interference with the equipment and the poor visibility of the patient once inside the magnet bore. A full discussion with the anaesthetist during the site planning stage should enable some of their difficulties to be overcome. For instance, piped gases in the scanning room are a major advantage and should be installed during construction.

The anaesthetic machine, monitoring devices, all tubing and attachments need to be non-magnetic and compatible with the system. Non-ferrous anaesthetic machines and patient monitoring systems are now available and, although costly, are essential.

The problem of the depth of the magnet bore preventing good visual monitoring of the patient can be overcome with a well-positioned light directed into the bore. Some manufacturers provide lighting built into the magnet bore.

A preparation/recovery area is essential and this allows intubation and anaesthetisation with the use of routine anaesthetic equipment to take place away from the scanning room. Once anaesthetised the patient can be transferred to the scanning room and, when the examination is complete, moved back to the recovery room to be awoken. This saves valuable scanning time as another patient can be brought straight in.

11 Applications and Pathology

There are a number of radiological texts available which cover a vast range of pathological conditions in great detail. It is our intention in this chapter to focus on the radiographic side of image acquisition and to illustrate some of the more common pathological conditions encountered.

The aim of any diagnostic imaging procedure is to detect any abnormality present, show its precise location and extent and, if possible, characterise the lesion. MRI is no exception. Its multiplanar facility gives extremely good anatomical definition and the superior soft tissue contrast obtained using the technique helps to differentiate the components and extent of a lesion. Unfortunately, however, MRI cannot be specific in diagnosing the particular type of lesion as precise tissue characterisation by T1 and T2 values is unreliable. The use of intravenous contrast media has proved useful in further detection of lesions as well as giving more accurate information regarding their true extent.

It is essential that the basic principles of MRI are understood in order to achieve the necessary tissue contrast (i.e. T1 or T2 weighting). There are numerous options available to reduce motion and artifacts and a knowledge of when and how to use them is essential. The choice of body, head or surface coil needs to be taken into consideration depending upon the area being imaged.

MRI is an evolving field, with new applications, hardware and software continually being developed. It is therefore difficult to give precise guidelines regarding pulse sequences and parameters as they vary according to the capabilities of different scanners. Imaging parameters such as field of view (FOV), number of signal averages (NSA) and matrix size must be modified to give optimal signal in an acceptable scanning time, and an understanding of the interrelationships of the imaging parameters is required.

The reconstruction matrix is important in image resolution. The larger the number of pixels per unit area the better the resolution of the images; the trade-off, however, is the scanning time and signal-to-noise ratio (SNR). Thicker slices (larger voxels) will give an improved SNR but partial volume effects may obscure fine structures or lesions, so reducing resolution. A compromise is therefore necessary between SNR and spatial resolution in order to keep the scanning time acceptable. The matrix selected in the frequency-encoding direction is usually kept at a high value (256). The number of views in the phase-encoding direction, which controls the acquisition time, can be reduced within reason to keep imaging time as short as possible; this results in a proportionate reduction in resolution in the phase-encoding direction.

The aspects of MRI that cause radiographers most concern are probably selection of the most appropriate pulse sequence for demonstrating the pathology and the plane in which to perform the sequence. Patients present for MRI with specific symptoms and a provisional diagnosis from the referring clinician. This gives a good indication to the radiographer or radiologist of precisely where to scan and, in conjunction with any accompanying previous radiographs, allows a plan for the examination to be made. We have tried here to give an overview of pulse sequences and parameters to allow an understanding of how and why they are used.

As with any aspect of radiography, positioning of the patient is important and it is beneficial to have the patient straight and in a true anatomical position. Foam pads and straps will help to immobilise the patient. However, since MRI can be a lengthy procedure it is better to have the patient comfortable and still than perfectly positioned and moving. It is always possible in MRI to compensate for the patient's position by using pilots in all three planes if necessary from which true anatomical scanning planes can be prescribed.

In this chapter we will consider the various anatomical areas in turn under the following headings: (1) technical considerations, (2) patient positioning, (3) pulse sequences, (4) scanning planes, (5) contrast enhancement, (6) problem areas and (7) new improved techniques.

THE BRAIN

Technical Considerations

All scanners have dedicated coils which are used to image the brain. These are usually quadrature transmit/receive coils of a "helmet" configuration.

Patient Positioning

The patient is positioned supine in the head coil and immobilised in a comfortable position.

Pulse Sequences

Spin echo pulse sequences are usually used when imaging the brain. T2-weighted sequences are most sensitive to pathology and should be acquired in the most suitable plane. Usually a multiple spin echo sequence is chosen. A shorter echo time (TE) of, for example, 25 ms gives proton density information whilst a longer TE of 80–100 ms gives T2 information. The proton density image is useful for assessing periventricular pathology such as multiple sclerosis, as the hyperintense plaques are visible against the hypointense cerebrospinal fluid (CSF).

An alternative to the first echo proton density weighted sequence is a "mildly" T2-weighted image using an intermediate TE of 40–60 ms. Images produced in this way have very little contrast between the different tissues allowing better visualisation of small periventricular lesions.

The inversion recovery sequence can be used to produce a variety of different types of contrast.

1. *STIR: Short Tau (Time) Inversion Recovery.* By nullifying the signal from fat (using a TI of around 100 ms – the precise figure varies according to field strength) certain pathological information can be gained from this sequence regarding lipomas or optic nerve disease.

2. *Medium TI.* These images show heavily T1-weighted contrast for very good anatomical detail and excellent differentiation between the grey and white matter of the brain (TI 250–700 ms).

3. *Long TI (FLAIR): FLuid Attenuated Inversion Recovery Sequence.* The combination of a very long TR (6000 ms) and TI (1800–3000 ms) and a long TE (150–200 ms) has the effect of nullifying the signal from fluid, which in the brain is CSF. This effect can be utilised to produce T2-weighted images of tissues other than CSF, enabling better definition of small periventricular lesions that could otherwise be masked. Because CSF is a slowly flowing fluid nullifying its signal produces an added advantage of reducing artifacts within the image.

Gradient echo pulse sequences are not routinely used when imaging the brain due to their sensitivity to susceptibility effects at air/bone/brain interfaces (mastoid air cells, sphenoid sinuses). In certain instances this fact can be used, however, to aid in diagnosis as the increased sensitivity of the sequence can detect calcification, flow and haemorrhage. The gradient echo scan enhances the magnetic susceptibility effect of acute and chronic haemorrhage which allows easier visualisation.

Scanning Planes

Images are usually acquired in all three orthogonal planes. Initially a sagittal T1-weighted (short TR/TE) sequence is performed using a 5 mm slice thickness and 10% slice gap (to prevent cross-talk). To include the entire head a FOV of 22–25 cm is used.

The sagittal plane will give useful information about midline structures such as the corpus callosum, sella and third ventricle, and also the brain stem, fourth ventricle and aqueduct.

A T2-weighted sequence is performed in the most suitable plane; usually the axial plane is chosen because of the direct correlation with CT scans. The midline sagittal slice can be used to prescribe the axial sequence, angling it parallel to the hard palate as shown in Fig. 11.1

A coronal sequence prescribed from the midline sagittal slice angled parallel to the brain stem (Fig. 11.2) can be used to highlight periventricular or corpus callosum abnormalities as well as lesions at the vertex and the temporal lobe. When examining a patient with temporal lobe epilepsy for mesial temporal sclerosis (Fig. 11.3), it is very important to maintain symmetry by scanning in the true orthogonal planes (multiplanar pilots are necessary).

A slice thickness of 5–7 mm is sufficient to image the brain with a 1 mm slice gap. The T2-weighted sequence, however, requires a larger slice gap (20%) to prevent cross-talk.

The matrix size selected reflects the in-plane resolution (along with the FOV) and, with the high efficiency of modern head coils, a high-resolution image is desirable. This can be achieved with a 256 matrix (a reduction in phase-encoding views may be used to reduced overall scanning time).

Imaging the posterior fossa will require thinner slices in the region of 3–5 mm with a 10% slice gap.

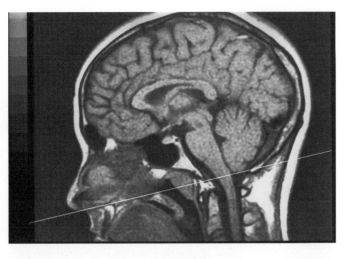

Fig. 11.1. SE T1-weighted sagittal midline slice through the brain showing the angle parallel to the hard palate used to prescribe the axial sequence.

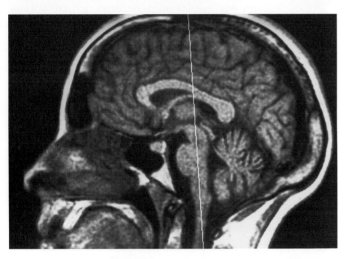

Fig. 11.2. SE T1-weighted sagittal midline slice through the brain showing the angle parallel to the brain stem used to prescribe the coronal sequence.

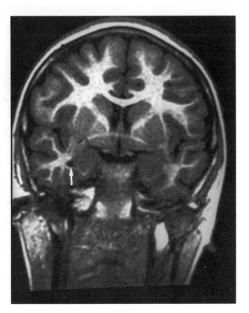

Fig. 11.3. Coronal T1-weighted IR sequence (TR 2000 ms, TI 600 ms, TE 30 ms) of the brain demonstrating temporal mesial sclerosis (*arrow*). By undertaking multiple plane pilots symmetry is achieved, which is very important in demonstrating these subtle lesions.

This reduces the partial volume effect within the slice at the expense of a reduction in the SNR. However, when considering the anatomical region under investigation the improved resolution of the images outweighs the reduction in SNR and therefore image quality. A smaller FOV of 20 cm will further improve resolution when combined with a suitable matrix (i.e. 256).

Contrast Medium

Intravenous contrast medium has been used for a number of years for diseases of the central nervous system (CNS). Like X-ray contrast media it penetrates areas of breakdown in the blood–brain barrier. There is no doubt that it has increased the sensitivity, specificity and accuracy of MRI in the brain. Oedema and tumour are often very difficult to separate but the use of i.v. contrast medium has made this possible. When i.v. contrast has been used T1-weighted sequences will show any pathology as areas of enhancement (Fig. 11.4).

Problem Areas

Specialised techniques for reducing motion artifacts on the images such as peripheral gating and flow compensation (gradient moment nulling), can play a part in effectively reducing ghost artifacts from CSF flow. Presaturation slabs applied below the scanning plane can be used to reduce vascular motion artifacts and have a role to play in the detection of flow.

In the axial plane the phase-encoding axis should be swapped from the Y (anteroposterior) to the X (left to right) axis to prevent orbital motion causing artifacts in the posterior fossa.

New Improved Techniques

The fast spin echo technique allows a 512 reconstruction matrix to be used for further increased resolution (Fig. 11.5). Alternatively if used with a "normal" matrix (256) it allows a second plane of T2-weighted images to be performed in an acceptable time.

Three-dimensional volume acquisition allows multiplanar reconstructions, so anatomical information can be obtained from one acquisition and retrospectively reformatted as required. The thin slices used also provide greater resolution and fewer partial volume effects. Fast spoiled or magnetisation prepared gradient echo sequences are usually employed, producing T1 weighting and keeping scanning times acceptable (Fig. 11.6).

Angiography sequences can be used to detect flow, check vascular patency, and demonstrate aneurysms and arteriovenous malformations.

CSF flow studies not only demonstrate flow but also quantify it. This can be useful in assessing hydrocephalus and its causes.

Perfusion studies using bolus contrast injections are now being used for the further evaluation of cranial tumours.

Diffusion weighted imaging sequences are sensitive to the molecular motion produced by diffusion and

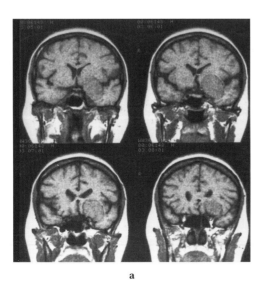
a

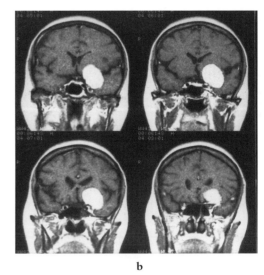
b

Fig. 11.4   a SE TI-weighted sequence (TR 450 ms, TE 21 ms) of the brain in the coronal plane. The lesion is not easily seen although the distortion of the ventricles on the left side indicates its presence. **b** The same patient using the same parameters but after the administration of i.v. contrast medium. The lesion (meningioma) can easily be seen as an area of high signal intensity.

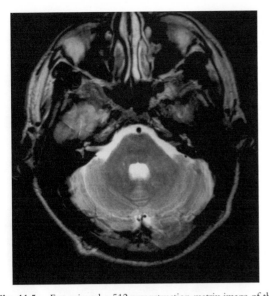

Fig. 11.5. Fast spin echo 512 reconstruction matrix image of the brain showing the obvious increase in image resolution when using this technique (TR 4000, effective TE 85 ms, NSA 4, acquisition time 6 min 24 s). (Courtesy of IGE Medical Systems.)

may prove to have increased sensitivity for demonstrating early pathological changes.

Functional imaging allows the isolation and assessment of certain centres within the brain according to their function (e.g. visual centres in the occipital lobe).

Pathology

A comprehensive review of the different types of pathology of the brain is beyond the scope of this text, and there are already many fine volumes on the subject. We have, however, included here some examples of the most common pathology found in the brain.

Before considering the abnormal appearances of the brain we will first consider its normal appearance. Table 11.1 shows the MRI appearances of different tissues according to the weighting of the pulse sequence selected (i.e. T1, T2, proton density).

Tumours of the brain can be divided into intra-axial

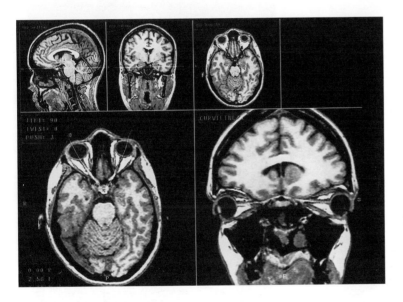

Fig. 11.6. Multiplanar reconstructions of the brain from a single T1-weighted three-dimensional spoiled gradient echo sequence. Isotrophic voxels allow high-quality multiplanar images to be obtained. (Courtesy of Picker International Ltd.)

Table 11.1. The MRI appearances of the brain and associated structures

	T1 weighted	Proton density	T2 weighted
Cortical bone	No signal	No signal	No signal
Fatty marrow	Hyperintense	Hyperintense	Isointense
Fat	Hyperintense	Hyperintense	Isointense
Air	Hypointense	Hypointense	Hypointense
White matter	Isointense/hypointense	Isointense/hypointense	Isointense/hypointense
Grey matter	Isointense/hyperintense	Isointense/hyperintense	Isointense/hyperintense
Muscle	Isointense	Isointense	Isointense
Flowing blood (rapid)	Hypointense	Hypointense	Hypointense
Flowing blood (slow)	Isointense	Isointense	Hyperintense
Cerebrospinal fluid	Hypointense	Isointense	Hyperintense

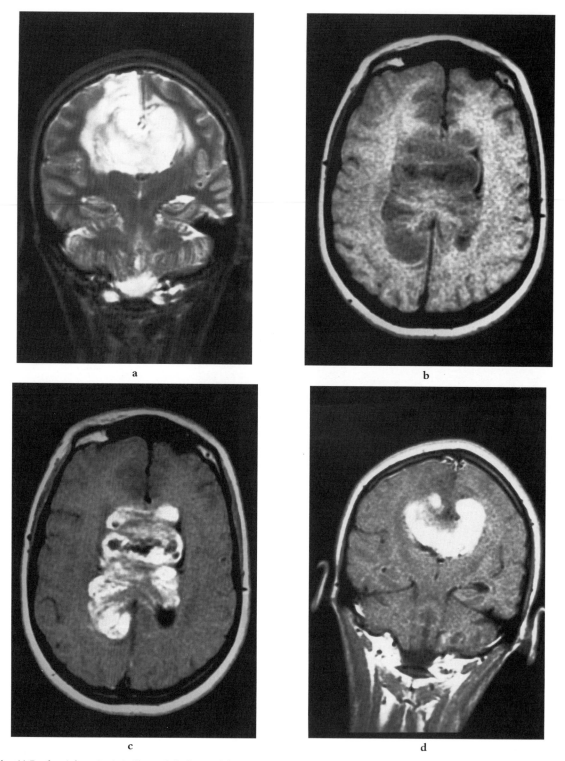

Fig. 11.7a–d. A large intrinsic "butterfly" glioma of the corpus callosum. **a** Coronal SE T2-weighted image (TR 480 ms, TE 21 ms) which shows the lesion and surrounding oedema as an area of high signal intensity. **b** Axial SE T1-weighted image (TR 480 ms, TE 21 ms) showing the obvious abnormality. **c** Axial SE T1-weighted image (TR 480 ms, TE 21 ms) after i.v. contrast medium showing the enhancing areas of the lesion and therefore its true extent. **d** Post-contrast coronal SE T1-weighted image (same parameters) helps to define further the real extent of the lesion.

(intrinsic) and extra-axial (extrinsic). The ability to distinguish between these two types is crucial as the degree of malignancy is much higher in intra-axial tumours. MRI allows this distinction to be made much easier than any other imaging modality (Figs. 11.7, 11.8). Tumours often have surrounding oedema and a high degree of oedema usually indicates a more aggressive tumour. MRI is very sensitive in demonstrating oedema, particularly on T2-weighted sequences where it can be seen as a high signal (Fig. 11.9).

Infections

MRI can detect lesions earlier than CT and can therefore be useful in localising infections.

CNS infections may represent a primary process (e.g. meningitis, encephalitis, abscess) or be part of a systemic disease. Bacterial meningitis and ventriculitis result in meningeal or ependymal enhancement on MRI similar to that on CT, but earlier and more easily visualised with coronal sections. MRI is extremely sensitive to early oedematous changes produced by viral encephalitis, especially that associated with herpes simplex infection, allowing earlier treatment.

Enhancement may be seen with cerebritis and abscess formation. Toxoplasmosis and lymphoma demonstrate enhancement whereas in AIDS patients non-enhancing lesions are sometimes due to progressive multifocal leucoencephalopathy (PML) or cytomegalovirus (CMV).

Demyelinating Diseases

The commonest demyelinating disease is multiple sclerosis (MS). MRI cannot give a definitive diagnosis of MS as appearances can mimic other diseases (e.g. sarcoidosis, leucodystrophies and vascular abnormalities), but is used to confirm the presence of white matter lesions and to rule out any other pathology. Optic neuritis is a common feature of MS and therefore STIR (or an alternative fat suppression technique) is used to identify optic nerve lesions. For the brain the T2-weighted sequence (usually in the axial plane) shows lesions present in the periventricular and deep white matter regions (Fig. 11.10). Demyelination can also occur in the spinal cord and patients often present with spinal sensory loss, which necessitates imaging the spinal cord also. Acute demyelination causes a breakdown in the blood–brain barrier and acute MS plaques show enhancement on T1-weighted sequences following administration of i.v. contrast medium.

Intracranial Haemorrhage

The MRI appearances of haemorrhage are very confusing and for this reason it is worth considering the processes which occur during the breakdown of a haematoma. It is reasonable to expect that since haemoglobin contains iron it will influence the appearance of an evolving haematoma.

The evolving haematoma goes through several biochemical and pathological changes each of which has a different appearance on MRI depending on the pattern of the breakdown products of oxyhaemoglobin, deoxyhaemoglobin, methaemoglobin, hemichromes and haemosiderin. Whether these are intracellular or extracellular and intraparenchymal or extraparenchymal also plays an important role. The field strength, pulse sequence and stage/age of the haemorrhage all result in different MRI appearances that are based upon the concentration and changing magnetic properties of iron.

Intracerebral (Intraparenchymal) Haemorrhage

We will consider here the appearances of haemorrhage using spin echo T1- and T2-weighted images, although it is worth remembering the value of the gradient echo sequence due to its greater sensitivity to magnetic susceptibility.

Haemoglobin alternates between an oxygenated state (from lungs to tissues) and a deoxygenated state (from the tissues to the lungs). The iron in haemoglobin has to be in the reduced ferrous state in order to bind oxygen reversibly. However, when the red blood cell is trapped in a haematoma the haemoglobin converts into an oxidised form called methaemoglobin in which the iron is in a non-functional ferric state. Methaemoglobin is then transformed into other derivatives called hemichromes.

During the hyperacute stage (up to 24 hours), the haematoma is formed by oxyhaemoglobin and deoxyhaemoglobin within the intact red blood cells. In the acute stage (24 hours to 4 days), the haematoma is fomed primarily of deoxyhaemoglobin within the intact red blood cells. In the subacute stage (4 to 30 days), the deoxyhaemoglobin transforms into methaemoglobin, first at the periphery and then at the centre. After 10 days a resorption granuloma organises at the periphery of the haematoma; this is formed of macrophages which remove the iron from the haemoglobin. This iron forms the peripheral rim of haemosiderin (Fig. 11.11). The chronic stage is defined as from 30 days onwards. It is useful when describing the evolution of a haematoma to use well-defined stages, but it is important to remember that

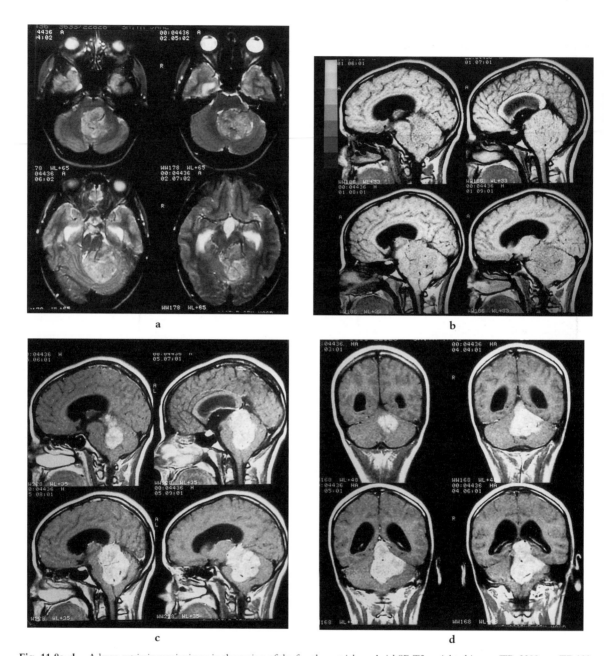

a

b

c

d

Fig. 11.8a–d. A large extrinsic meningioma in the region of the fourth ventricle. **a** Axial SE T2-weighted image (TR 2300 ms, TE 100 ms) showing a large lesion with mass effect distorting the normal brain tissues. The absence of high signal around the lesion (oedema) indicates it to be slow growing. **b** Sagittal SE T1-weighted image (TR 480 ms, TE 21 ms) shows a large lesion in the posterior fossa but its margins are indistinct. **c, d** Sagittal and coronal SE T1-weighted images respectively (same parameters) after i.v. contrast medium enhancement of the lesion, demonstrating its true extent.

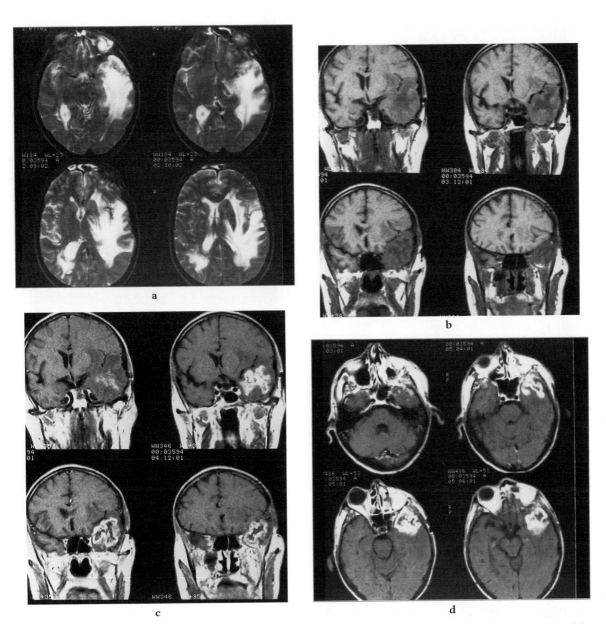

Fig. 11.9 a Axial SE T2-weighted images (TR 2300 ms, TE 100 ms) show marked high signal intensity throughout the whole of the temporal lobe, indicating a fast-growing lesion. Its precise localisation is very difficult (owing to the extensive oedema present. **b** Coronal SE T1-weighted images (TR 480 ms, TE 21 ms) show abnormal low signal within the temporal lobe (oedema). **c, d** Coronal and axial SE T1-weighted images respectively after i.v. contrast medium show the precise localisation of the lesion and the degree of oedema surrounding it. The differential diagnosis is metastases or radiation necrosis.

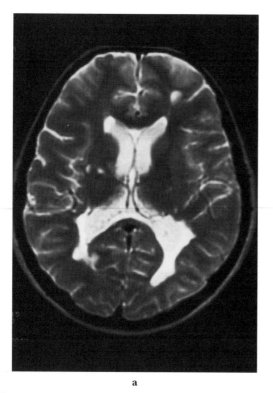
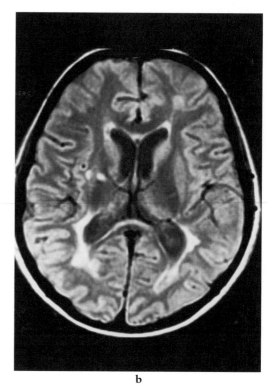

a   b

Fig. 11.10   a Axial SE T2-weighted images (TR 2300 ms, TE 100 ms) of the brain showing extensive high signal abnormalities throughout the white matter (chronic MS). **b** Axial proton density weighted images (TR 2300 ms, TE 25 ms) of the same patient at the same slice
locations help to demonstrate better the extent of the periventricular lesions.

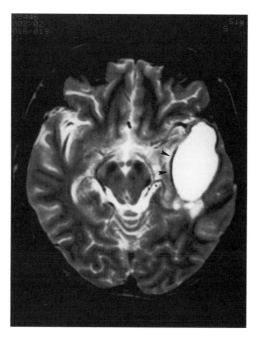

Fig. 11.11.   Axial SE T2-weighted image (TR 480 ms, TE 21 ms) of
the brain showing a large resolving intraparenchymal haematoma. The
low-signal rim of haemosiderin can be seen (*arrows*) around the high
signal of the methaemoglobin. (Courtesy of IGE Medical Systems.)

these stages all coexist, the different layers of the haematoma being at different stages of evolution.

Table 11.2 demonstrates the signal intensity changes which take place in the various stages of an intracerebral haematoma. By using suitable sequences each stage can be highlighted, which is very useful in subacute and chronic lesions when CT is non-specific.

Hyperacute subarachnoid haemorrhage cannot be demonstrated using MRI and CT remains the investigation of choice. In the subacute stage methaemoglobin is formed, resulting in an increase in signal intensity on T1-weighted sequences. These appearances are further complicated in mild subarachnoid haemorrhage by the fact that resorption of red blood cells may occur before methaemoglobin formation. Aneurysms and arteriovenous malformations are demonstrated by the signal void produced in the vessels by flowing blood (Fig. 11.12), adherent clot or adjacent brain oedema. MR angiography sequences will, as their sensitivity improves, have an important role to play in the evaluation of patients with aneurysms and arteriovenous malformations.

Head Injury

MRI can be used in the evaluation of head injuries. However, the inability to monitor critically ill patients easily in the MRI scanner can present problems. CT scanning is a more practical alternative.

Subdural and Extradural Haematomas

Subdural and extradural haematomas evolve in a simi-lar manner to intracerebral haematomas with one exception: the transport of iron away from the haematoma occurs much more rapidly and so the characteristic rim of signal loss due to haemosiderin and ferritin is no longer present.

The anatomical distortion associated with these haematomas can easily be detected with the multiplanar facility of MRI. The absence of bone artifacts aids in the detection of small haematomas. Scanning in the coronal and axial plane best demonstrates these lesions and can help to differentiate between the two (Fig. 11.13).

Contusion and Shearing Injuries

MRI can help in the evaluation of contusion and shearing injuries but CT remains the primary investigation of choice in the acutely ill patient (Fig. 11.14).

Infarction

Since MRI is sensitive to oedema it is well suited to detecting infarction and can show abnormal findings as early as 2–4 hours after vessel occlusion. MRI is useful in identifying infarcts in the brain stem and lower posterior fossa (Fig. 11.15), which can cause problems in CT due to the artifacts produced by the surrounding bone.

The classic pattern of cerebral infarction is a wedge-shaped abnormality involving the cortex and variable amounts of the subcortical tissue. Haemorrhage into infarcts represents the blood oozing from the damaged capillaries and is demonstrated as a cortical ribbon of

Table 11.2. The spin echo MRI appearances of intracerebral haematomas

Stage of haemorrhage	Signal intensity (relative to grey matter)	
	T1	T2
Hyperacute (<24 hours)	Isointense	Isointense
Acute (1–4 days)	Hypointense	Hypointense
Subacute (4–7 days)	Hyperintense	Hypointense
Subacute (7–30 days)	Hyperintense	Hyperintense
Chronic[a] (>30 days)		
Rim	Isointense	Hypointense
Centre	Hyperintense	Hyperintense

[a] The appearances of chronic haematoma change with time and cannot be categorised simply.

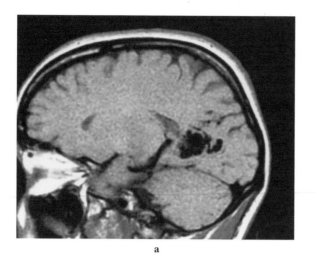

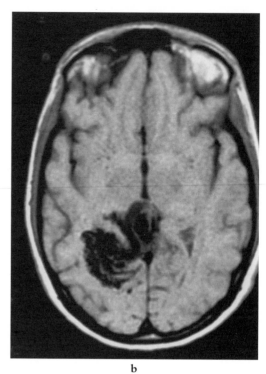

Fig. 11.12a,b. Sagittal and axial SE T1-weighted images respectively (TR 480 ms, TE 21 ms) of the brain demonstrating an occipital arteriovenous malformation. There are characteristic signal voids present from the fast-flowing arteriovenous shunts. (Courtesy of Siemens.)

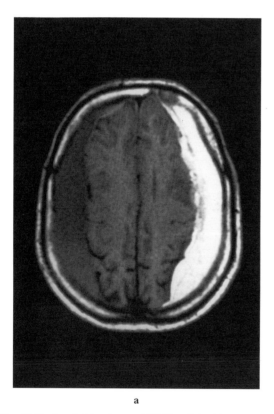

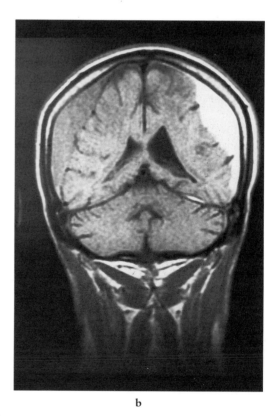

Fig. 11.13a,b. Axial and coronal SE T1-weighted images respectively (TR 480 ms, TE 21 ms) of the brain demonstrating bilateral subdural haematomas in different stages of evolution.

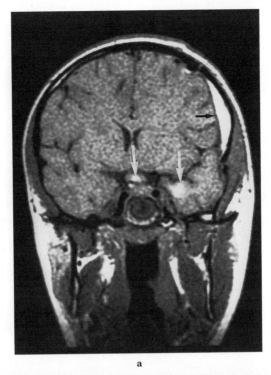

a

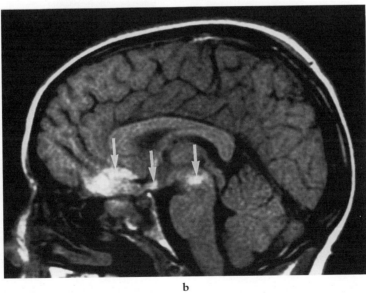

b

Fig. 11.14 a Coronal SE T1-weighted image (TR 480 ms, TE 21 ms) of the brain demonstrating an extradural haematoma (*black arrow*) and contusions (*white arrows*). **b** Sagittal T1-weighted midline slice showing contusion in the frontal lobe, chiasm and midbrain (*arrows*).

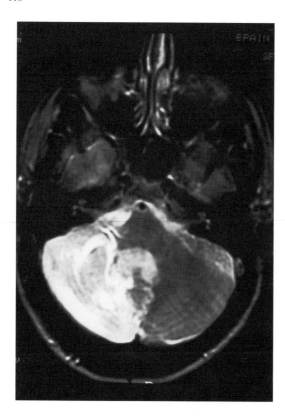

Fig. 11.15. Axial SE T2-weighted image (TR 2300 ms, TE 100 ms) of the brain demonstrating infarction of the whole of the right side of the cerebellum.

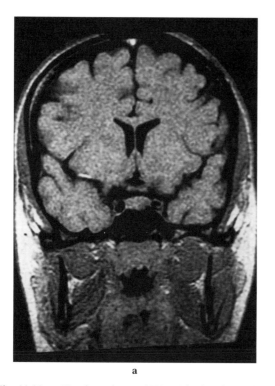

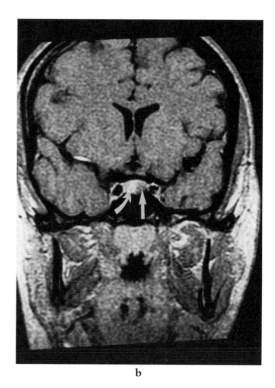

a   b

Fig. 11.16 **a** Unenhanced coronal T1-weighted gradient echo (GRASS) image (TR 300 ms, flip angle 75°, TE 12 ms) of the pituitary gland. Following i.v. contrast medium the normal pituitary gland enhances (*curved arrow*), strongly confirming the presence of a microadenoma (*straight arrow*).

low or high signal depending on the pulse sequence selected and the stage of the haemorrhage. Old infarcts have a more complex signal pattern.

A flow void is usually present in the main cerebral arteries with spin echo imaging. This flow void disappears in cases of arterial occlusion or slow flow. The use of gradient echo techniques, which are more susceptible to flow, will confirm this one way or the other. MRI can also detect lack of venous flow (venous sinus thrombosis); once detected this allows observation of occlusion following treatment. Again the gradient echo sequence is more sensitive in the detection of flow.

Administration of i.v. contrast medium may help to distinguish infarct from an infectious process or tumour.

Imaging of Different Regions of the Brain

Sellar/Parasellar Region

Technical Considerations

The head coil can be used to image the sellar/parasellar region.

Patient Positioning

The patient is positioned supine in the head coil and immobilised in a comfortable position.

Pulse Sequences

Spin echo pulse sequences are usually used to image the sellar region.

2DFT gradient echo pulse sequences suffer from susceptibility artifacts in the sellar region and are therefore not routinely employed, although 3DFT gradient echo pulse sequence techniques with short TE times and small voxels are more commonly used (see New Improved Techniques below).

Scanning Planes

Multiplanar MRI accurately defines the full extent of sellar/parasellar lesions.

Sagittal and coronal planes are most useful in this region. When looking for small microadenomas a slice thickness of 2–3 mm allows visualisation of small lesions which could be obscured by partial volume effects if thicker slices were used. Similarly a small FOV (15–20 cm) and large reconstruction matrix (256) further aid high-resolution imaging.

T2-weighted images can be acquired in the coronal plane to aid visualisation of the pituitary gland and its relationship to the cerebral blood vessels in the para-/suprasellar region.

Contrast Enhancement

The normal pituitary gland can have a characteristic area of high signal in the posterior lobe on T1-weighted images. After administration of i.v. contrast medium the normal pituitary gland enhances, the posterior lobe enhancing a few seconds before the anterior lobe. Dynamic contrast studies have revealed changes in this normal pattern of enhancement in certain pathological conditions.

Using routine T1-weighted sequences after intravenous contrast medium, microadenomas show delayed enhancement compared with the normal gland (Fig. 11.16). Macroadenomas show moderate or marked enhancement which helps to define the margins of the tumour and reveal the extent of involvement of the surrounding structures (carotid arteries, optic chiasm, etc.) (Fig. 11.17). Parasellar and suprasellar lesions such as meningiomas, chiasmatic/hypothalamic tumours and craniopharyngiomas (Fig. 11.18) are more accurately defined using i.v. contrast medium.

Problem Areas

Because of the location of the sella, CSF flow and, more particularly, vascular flow can be a source of artifacts when imaging the pituitary region. Peripheral gating, gradient moment nulling and especially presaturation can be used to minimise these artifacts.

New Improved Techniques

Three-dimensional volume acquisition can be a useful additional sequence in the pituitary. The ability to obtain thin sequential slices is a major advantage of the technique (Fig. 11.19).

The fast spin echo sequence allows the acquisition of thinner T2-weighted images which will increase the sensitivity of the technique.

MR angiography sequences allow visualisation of the circle of Willis and other related vascular structures.

The use of perfusion imaging in the gland has already been mentioned. No doubt as the faster sequences become readily available it will be a feature of all pituitary examinations.

Internal Auditory Meatus

MRI is the modality of choice in most centres for imaging the posterior fossa, cerebellopontine angle (CPA) and internal auditory meatus (IAM), although CT is still required to image the bone detail of the middle ear. In MRI the lack of artifact from the bone, the multiplanar facilities and the use of thin slices allow the cranial nerves to be visualised with and without the administration of contrast media in order to detect any abnormalities.

Technical Considerations

The head coil is used when scanning the IAM.

Patient Positioning

The patient is positioned supine with the head in the head coil and immobilised in a comfortable position.

Pulse Sequences

The spin echo sequence is usually used. Many centres examine the IAM only with T1-weighted images, both with and without contrast.

T1-weighted gradient echo sequences are an alternative to the spin echo sequence (being slightly faster), although there is still the slight problem of susceptibility. T2-weighted sequences may sometimes be beneficial, especially in demonstrating cystic portions of any lesions.

Scanning Planes

Axial and coronal planes best demonstrate the IAM and the course of the VIIth and VIIIth cranial nerves.

When examining the IAM for small intracanalicular neuromas a very high resolution is required, and hence a slice thickness of 2–3 mm is used for the T1-weighted sequences. A 20 cm FOV and a reconstruction matrix of 256 will produce high in-plane resolution.

Contrast Enhancement

Intravenous contrast medium is routinely used to confirm or exclude the presence of an acoustic neuroma. Small intracanalicular lesions may not be seen on unenhanced scans. The true extent of larger lesions is also better demonstrated using contrast (Figs. 11.20 and 11.21).

Problem Areas

Vascular flow can be a problem in the posterior fossa, the transverse sinuses often causing artifacts when i.v. contrast medium has been used due to the increased signal from the slow-flowing blood. Flow compensation can be used to minimise this effect; this results in the use of a slightly longer TE time. Presaturation may also be used to minimise the artifact further.

New Improved Techniques

Fast spin echo allows 3 mm T2-weighted images to be acquired and, if used in conjunction with a 512 reconstruction matrix, enables the production of very high resolution images. Images of such great detail will allow visualisation of the entire course of the nerves from brain stem to cochlea.

Orbits

The superior anatomical detail of the orbital structures that is achieved in conjunction with the multiplanar imaging facility makes MRI a valuable modality for evaluating orbital lesions.

Technical Considerations

Dedicated surface coils are now available from most manufacturers for examining the orbits. These are usually of a goggle design allowing both orbits to be imaged simultaneously, visualising the optic nerves as far back as the chiasm. An alternative for those without dedicated coils is to use circular multi-purpose surface coils (3 inch for a single orbit or 5 inch for both orbits) in conjunction with the head coil to view as far back as the optic chiasm and beyond.

Patient Positioning

The patient is made as comfortable as possible and

immobilised in position. The surface coil or coils are positioned as close to the orbit as possible and the patient asked to keep the eyes still by focusing on a fixed point within the imager.

Pulse Sequences

The spin echo sequence is used when imaging the orbit. Most orbital tissue has relatively short T2 values resulting in marked signal reduction if very long TE times are used.

T1-weighted sequences are used in multiple planes with an appropriate plane being imaged with a T2-weighted sequence.

STIR is a useful additional sequence because it suppresses the signal from periorbital fat. Alternative fat suppression techniques such as chemical shift imaging and fat saturation can also be employed.

Scanning Planes

Slight modifications in technique will arise when scanning individual orbits. It is our experience that scanning both orbits simultaneously allows direct comparisons to be made.

Images are acquired in all three orthogonal planes. Sagittal images can be prescribed, angling along the optic nerves from the appropriate axial image.

A FOV of 15–20 cm in conjunction with a 256 reconstruction matrix gives high in-plane resolution and a slice thickness of 3 mm reduces partial volume effects.

A thin slice of T2-weighted sequence in the axial plane can be useful but the prolongation of the scanning time makes the image more prone to motion artifacts, as is the STIR sequence. For this reason either one or the other is performed. The STIR sequence is probably best obtained in the coronal plane, which accurately delineates the optic nerves and orbital muscles.

Contrast Enhancement

Contrast is not routinely used when imaging the orbits. However, it can be valuable in assessing MS plaques within the orbit when used in conjunction with a STIR sequence (negative enhancement) or a T1-weighted fat saturation sequence.

Problem Areas

Orbital motion is the main limiting factor of the tech-

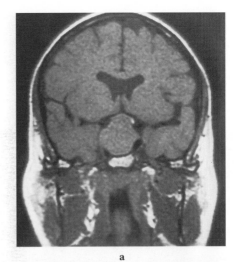

a

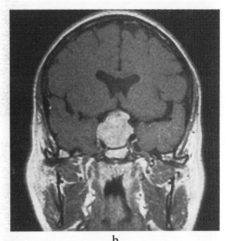

b

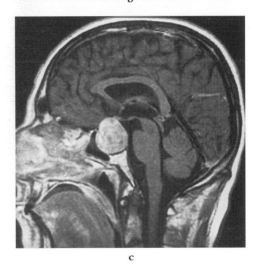

c

Fig. 11.17 a Coronal SE T1-weighted (TR 480 ms, TE 21 ms) unenhanced image showing a large hypointense lesion (macroadenoma) in the region of the pituitary. **b, c** Coronal and sagittal SE T1-weighted images respectively (TR 480 ms, TE 21 ms) after i.v. contrast medium showing enhancement of the lesion.

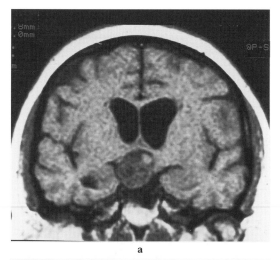

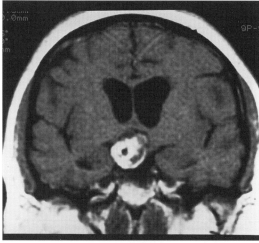

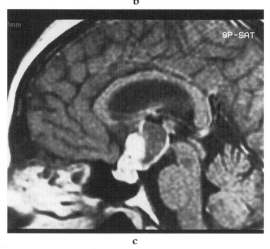

nique and so patient cooperation is vital.

The bright signal from periorbital fat can be a problem but different methods available to overcome this (STIR, chemical saturation, etc.) have already been discussed.

New Improved Techniques

Three-dimensional volume acquisition technique allows greater resolution and contiguous thinner slices.

The fast spin echo technique allows thin slice T2-weighted images to be acquired more quickly, thus reducing motion artifacts.

The fast inversion recovery sequence will allow STIR images to be obtained in a more acceptable acquisition time.

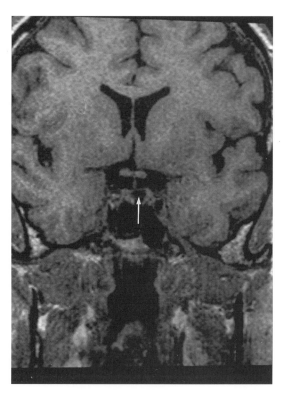

Fig. 11.18 **a** Coronal SE T1-weighted image (TR 480 ms, TE 21 ms) of the brain demonstrating a large hypointense cystic lesion. **b, c** Coronal and sagittal images respectively after i.v. contrast medium demonstrating strong enhancement of the lesion with some low signal areas which most probably represent calcification. The lesion was diagnosed as a craniopharyngioma.

Fig. 11.19. A three-dimensional gradient echo T1-weighted coronal image (TR 30 ms, flip angle 30°, TE 13 ms, slice thickness 1.5 mm) revealing a hypointense lesion (*arrow*) in the region of the pituitary gland diagnosed as a microadenoma. (Courtesy of Philips Medical Systems.)

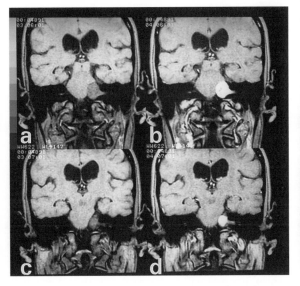

Fig. 11.20 a,c Coronal SE T1-weighted unenhanced images (TR 480 ms, TE 21 ms) demonstrating a large hypointense mass in the left cerebellopontine angle adjacent to the internal auditory meatus. **b, d** Coronal SE T1-weighted images (TR 450 ms, TE 21 ms) after i.v. contrast medium demonstrating the extent of the lesion and its extension into the internal auditory meatus that proves it to be an acoustic neuroma.

Fig. 11.21.   SE T1-weighted axial image (TR 450 ms, TE 21 ms) after intravenous contrast medium in the same patient as Fig. 11.20.

THE SPINE

MRI is the most effective method of imaging the spine and surrounding soft tissues and for many spinal disorders is now replacing CT and myelography as the imaging technique of choice. Disc protrusion, syrinxes, spinal cord compression, haemorrhage, contusion, metastatic deposits, marrow disorders and congenital malformations can all be readily visualised on MR images.

Although most MRI scanners have a body coil incorporated into the housing, images of the spine using the body coil are not of very good quality because the coil is too distant from the spine. A dedicated surface coil is essential for high-quality spinal images.

Table 11.3 lists the MRI appearances of the different spinal structures using a spin echo pulse sequence.

Common Scanning Parameters used in Spinal Imaging

Pulse Sequences

Spin echo sequences are commonly used when imag-

ing the spine. A multiple spin echo sequence can be used to produce proton density and T2-weighted images.

Gradient echo sequences are often preferred due to their ability to obtain a myelographic effect in a relatively short scanning time (compared with conventional spin echo T2). However, in the post-operative spine there are often metallic remnants left behind after surgery which cause susceptibility artifacts and so degrade the images. A spin echo sequence is less sensitive to these artifacts and would be preferable in a post-operative patient. The gradient echo pulse sequence can also be used to acquire T1-weighted images or phase difference images when looking for metastases (see Fig. 3.19, p.).

STIR is an alternative to phase difference imaging for highlighting metastatic changes. It can also be of some value in trauma cases to demonstrate areas of haemorrhage, but is dependent upon the condition of the patient.

Scanning Planes

The sagittal and parasagittal (T1-weighted) images give a good anatomical demonstration of the discs, spinal cord in longitudinal section and vertebral bodies. This is complemented by a T2-weighted sequence which demonstrates any pathological changes.

Table 11.3. MRI appearances of the spine and associated structures

	T1 weighted	Proton density	T2 weighted
Cortical bone	No signal	No signal	No signal
Fatty marrow	Hyperintense	Hyperintense	Isointense
Annulus			
Fibrosa	Isointense	Isointense	Hypointense
Pulposa	Isointense	Isointense	Hyperintense
Spinal cord	Isointense/hyperintense	Isointense/hyperintense	Isointense/hyperintense
Muscle	Isointense	Isointense	Isointense
Fat	Hyperintense	Hyperintense	Isointense
Flowing blood (rapid)	Hypointense	Hypointense	Hypointense
Flowing blood (slow)	Isointense	Isointense	Hyperintense
Cerebrospinal fluid	Hypointense	Isointense	Hyperintense

The axial plane demonstrates the spinal cord in cross-section and therefore any degree of cord compression, the intravertebral foramina, the neural arch and any paraspinal extension.

Imaging of Different Regions of the Spine

Cervical Spine

Technical Considerations

Surface coils are available which have been designed specifically for the cervical spine. They can be saddle-shaped, Helmholtz or of a quadrature design for use with superconducting magnets or a solenoid design for vertical field systems. They have an effective range extending from the posterior fossa down to T2/3, depending on their design.

Patient Positioning

The patient is comfortably positioned within the coil using restraints to minimise any possible motion of the head and neck.

Pulse Sequences and Scanning Planes

Sagittal T1- and T2-weighted sequences are prescribed from a coronal pilot using a spin echo (multiple echo) or gradient echo sequence. From the acquired images a series of axial T1- or T2*-weighted images are obtained angled through the disc space, using either a spin echo or gradient echo sequence.

A FOV of 25–30 cm, depending upon the sensitivity of the coil, is used for the sagittal plane. A slice thickness of 3–5 mm with a 256 reconstruction matrix will produce high-resolution images. A FOV of 15–20 cm with a 256 reconstruction matrix is adequate for the axial plane.

Sagittal oblique scans perpendicular to the intravertebral foramina are useful in evaluating lateral discs.

T2* axial scans are sometimes preferred owing to their ability to demonstrate high signal from CSF in the subarachnoid space around the nerve roots. This is important for the visualisation of subtle lateral disc protrusions (Fig. 11.22). Fig. 11.23 is an example of a large C5/6 disc protrusion causing spinal cord compression, with a smaller disc at C4/5.

Images with the neck flexed and extended can be of use in certain instances, such as the assessment of atlanto-axial instability in patients with rheumatoid arthritis. The sagittal plane demonstrates this most dramatically but the axial plane can also be useful when assessing the degree of cord compression (Fig. 11.24).

Contrast Enhancement

Intravenous contrast medium is administered for the further evaluation of intramedullary (Fig. 11.25), intradural (Fig. 11.26) and extradural lesions (Fig. 11.27).

Problem Areas

Swallowing is one of the major artifact problems encountered in the cervical spine. This can be overcome by the application of a presaturation pulse anteriorly or by swapping the direction of the phase-encoding axis (from anterior/posterior (X) to superior/inferior (Z)).

Another cause of artifacts in T2-weighted sequences of the cervical spine is CSF flow. This can be reduced by gradient moment nulling and/or peripheral gating. Gradient echo sequences use considerably shorter TE times than conventional T2-weighted spin echo sequences, resulting in reduced artifacts from CSF flow.

Aliasing (wraparound) can be encountered in axial sequences, especially in the lower cervical spine. Antialiasing techniques remove the artifacts from within the FOV.

New Improved Techniques

Three-dimensional volume imaging allowing multiplanar reformats. It is hoped that this technique will prove to be the gold standard when evaluating radiculopathy.

Fast spin echo allows T2-weighted sequences to be performed in a much shorter imaging time.

As previously mentioned, angiography coils have been developed to scan from the aortic arch to the circle of Willis. An unexpected bonus of these, when used in conjunction with a 512 matrix and fast spin echo technique, is the ability to image both the head and cervical spine at the same time (Fig. 11.28).

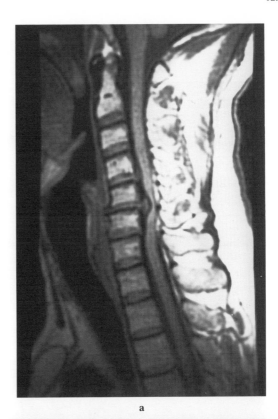

a

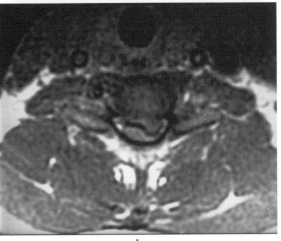

b

Fig. 11.23 **a** Sagittal SE T1-weighted sequence (TR 450 ms, TE 21 ms) of the cervical spine demonstrating a large disc protrusion at C5/6 causing compression of the spinal cord. There is also a small disc at C4/5 **b** Axial SE T1-weighted image (TR 450 ms, TE 21 ms). The disc lateralises to the left side and is compressing the spinal cord significantly.

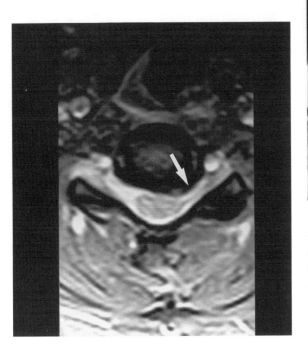

Fig. 11.22. Axial T2*-weighted gradient echo image (TR 450 ms, flip angle 30°, TE 20 ms) in the cervical spine demonstrating a subtle lateral disc protrusion (*arrow*).

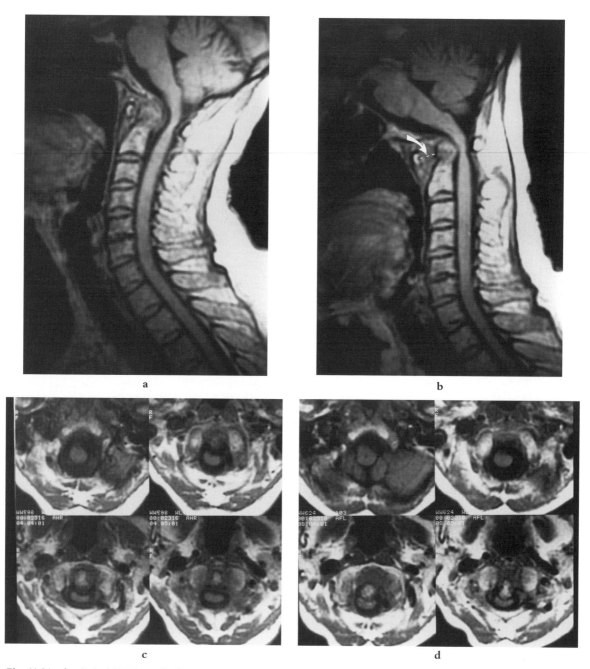

Fig. 11.24a–d. Sagittal SE T1-weighted image (TR 450 ms, TE 21 ms) of the cervical spine in extension (**a**) and flexion (**b**) demonstrating the degree of subluxation present. There is a marked increase in the distance between the anterior arch of the C1 and the odontoid peg (*arrow*) which is more apparent in the extension image. **c** Axial SE T1-weighted images (TR 450 ms, TE 21 ms) in extension (**c**) and flexion (**d**) showing the differing degrees of compression upon the spinal cord in the two positions.

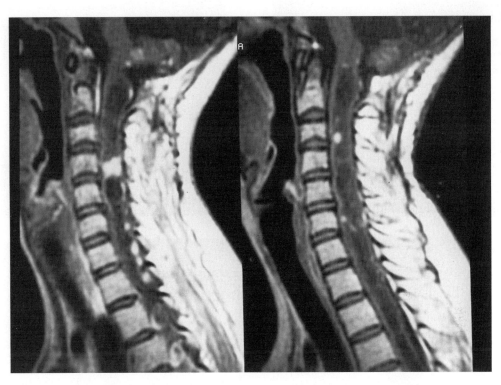

Fig. 11.25. Contrast-enhanced sagittal T1-weighted images (TR 450 ms, TE 21 ms) of the cervical spinal cord in a patient with known Von Hippel–Lindau syndrome. There is a large cystic cord with enhancing nodules present which represent multiple haemangiomas (intramedullary).

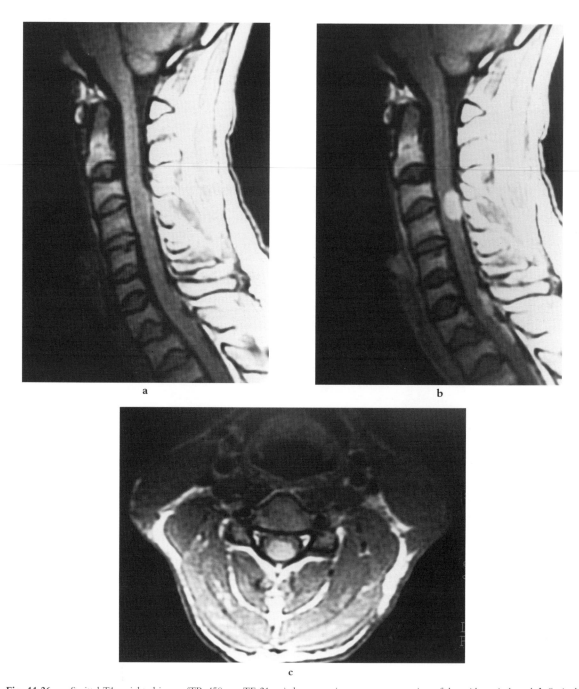

Fig. 11.26 **a** Sagittal T1-weighted image (TR 450 ms, TE 21 ms) demonstrating apparent expansion of the mid cervical cord. **b** Sagittal T1-weighted image (TR 450 ms, TE 21 ms) after i.v. contrast medium demonstrating multiple high signal abnormalities in the mid and lower cervical cord which are intradural but extramedullary. **c** Axial T1-weighted image (TR 500 ms, TE 21 ms) after i.v. contrast confirms the lesion to be extramedullary. These lesions were drop metastases from a cranial medulloblastoma.

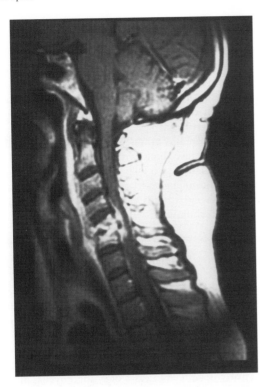

Fig. 11.27. Sagittal T1-weighted image (TR 450 ms, TE 21 ms) after i.v. contrast medium demonstrating an abnormal area of enhancement from the C5/6 vertebral bodies and discs and the extension of the abnormality into the neural canal causing cord compression.

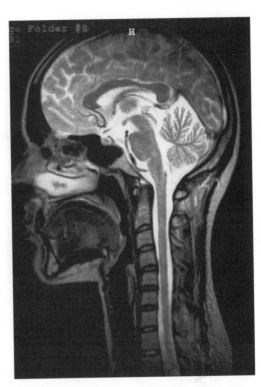

Fig. 11.28. Sagittal fast spin echo T2-weighted image (TR 5000 ms, TE 90 ms) using the angiographic coil in conjunction with a 512 reconstruction matrix, allowing both the brain and cervical spine to be imaged in one sequence. (Courtesy of Siemens.)

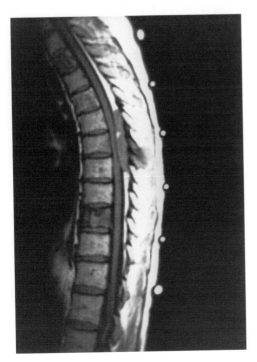

Fig. 11.29. Sagittal SE T1-weighted image (TR 450 ms, TE 21 ms) in the thoracic spine showing a metastatic deposit in the vertebral body with associated cord compression. The marking device attached to the patient's back allows direct localisation to the skin surface.

Thoracic Spine

Technical Considerations

Linear and quadrature surface coils are available for imaging of the thoracic and lumbar spine. Some manufacturers provide them in a movable bucky which allows easy adjustment of the coil position beneath the patient. This results in less manoeuvring of the patient if multiple areas of the spine are to be scanned.

Precise localisation of pathology to a particular vertebral level is important for the planning of surgery or radiotherapy. This can be achieved by acquiring a body coil image and counting lumbar up or cervical down, correlating them with the surface coil images. Alternatively a marking device fixed to the patient's skin can be visualised on the T1-weighted images, allowing direct localisation of a lesion to the skin surface (Fig. 11.29).

Patient Positioning

The patient is positioned supine and made as comfortable as possible. The centre of the coil is positioned to include the particular area of interest.

Pulse Sequences and Scanning Planes

Initially sagittal T1-weighted images are prescribed from a coronal pilot. A slice thickness of 3–5 mm in conjunction with a 30–35 cm FOV and 256 reconstruction matrix will give high in-plane resolution. The sagittal plane demonstrates well the entire length of the thoracic spinal cord.

A multiple spin echo sequence giving proton density and T2-weighted images is then performed in the sagittal plane.

An axial T1-weighted sequence is prescribed from the median sagittal section covering the area of interest using a 15–20 cm FOV, 3–5 mm slice thickness and 256 reconstruction matrix.

The coronal plane is not routinely used but can sometimes be very useful in cases of complex scoliosis or for improved visualisation of extra-axial lesions (Fig. 11.30).

Contrast Enhancement

The use of i.v. contrast medium in imaging the spine has improved both the sensitivity and specificity of MRI in the evaluation of spinal tumours (Fig. 11.31).

Problem Areas

Cardiac and respiratory motion can result in artifacts which substantially degrade the resultant images. Gating, respiratory compensation, presaturation slabs (applied anteriorly within the chest) and controlling the direction of the phase-encoding axis all help to reduce these artifacts.

CSF flow can also produce artifacts along the spinal cord which cause image degradation on the T2-weighted sequences. To help reduce these artifacts gradient moment nulling and a gating technique is applied.

Aliasing (wraparound) can be prevented by using antialiasing techniques.

New Improved Techniques

The fast spin echo sequence will allow T2-weighted images to be obtained in a much shorter acquisition time, which in turn will help to reduce motion artifacts.

Phased array coils are now available which allow the whole spine to be covered in one acquisition. This is particularly beneficial in cases of syringomyelia, multiple sclerosis and spinal drop metastases. The images are of a very high quality (Fig. 11.32).

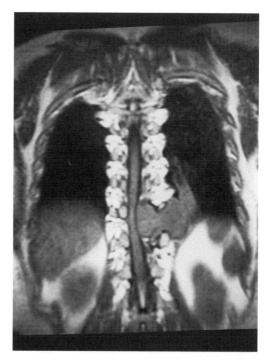

Fig. 11.30. Coronal SE T1-weighted image (TR 450 ms, TE 21 ms) showing a large soft tissue paraspinal mass extending through the neural foramen that was diagnosed as a neurofibroma.

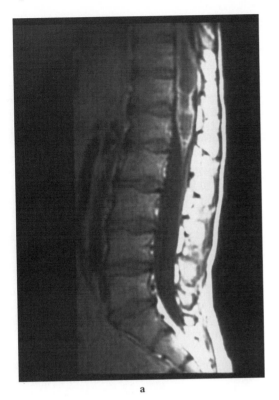

a

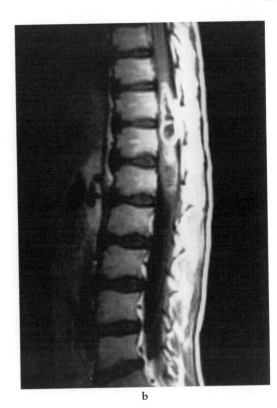

b

Fig. 11.31.a Sagittal SE T1-weighted image (TR 450 ms, TE 21 ms) demonstrating a large cystic lesion in the conus. **b** Sagittal SE T1-weighted images after i.v. contrast medium showing the true extent of the lesion, which was found to be an ependymoma.

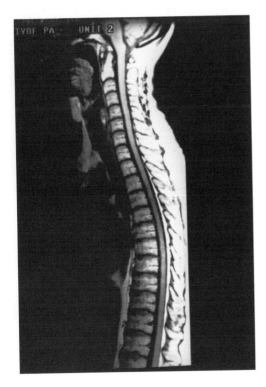

Fig. 11.32. Sagittal T1-weighted image (TR 800 ms, TE 23 ms, FOV 48 cm, 512 reconstruction matrix) demonstrating the whole spinal cord. (Courtesy of IGE Medical Systems.)

Lumbar Spine

Technical Considerations

As with the thoracic spine, a dedicated surface coil is used for the lumbar spine. An alternative is to use a 5 inch circular coil and examine the particular vertebral levels of interest (say L5/S1). The greater SNR of the smaller coil means that higher resolution can be obtained.

Patient Positioning

The patient is positioned supine with the lower costal margin at the centre of the surface coil and made as comfortable as possible. (If a smaller circular coil is used then it is positioned below the area of interest.)

Pulse Sequences and Scanning Planes

Initially sagittal T1-weighted images are prescribed from a coronal pilot. A slice thickness of 4–5 mm in conjunction with a 25–30 cm FOV and 256 reconstruction matrix will give high in-plane resolution.

A multiple spin echo sequence giving proton density and T2-weighted images is then performed in the sagittal plane.

An axial T1-weighted sequence is prescribed from the median sagittal section covering the area of interest using a 4–5 mm slice thickness, 15–20 cm FOV and 256 reconstruction matrix.

Fig. 11.33 is an example of a large central disc protrusion at L4/5 causing nerve root compression.

The coronal plane is rarely used although it can sometimes be helpful when demonstrating extra-axial lesions (e.g. neurofibroma, psoas abscess).

Contrast Enhancement

The use of i.v. contrast medium in imaging the spine has improved both the sensitivity and specificity of MRI in the evaluation of spinal tumours (Fig. 11.34).

In the post-operative spine intravenous contrast medium can help to differentiate fibrosis from recurrent disc (see Fig. 8.4, p. 86). Technique is critical when examining the post-operative spine. Axial and sagittal images are acquired after contrast and it is essential that the tuning factors (the attenuation or receive gain in particular) remain the same as for the pre-contrast series, allowing accurate assessment of enhancement around the nerve roots.

Problem Areas

Vascular artifacts and abdominal motion can be a problem. Presaturation slabs (anteriorly) will minimise these. Signal averaging will also reduce them but at the expense of increased scanning time.

CSF flow is not so much of a problem as in the thoracic spine, but in our experience gradient moment nulling is still of benefit for the multiple spin echo sequence.

Aliasing (wraparound) can be prevented by using antialiasing techniques.

New Improved Techniques

The fast spin echo sequence allows a reduction in scanning time for T2-weighted images. Axial T2-weighted images are proving to be a useful additional sequence when evaluating nerve roots, particularly in the case of arachnoiditis (Fig. 11.35).

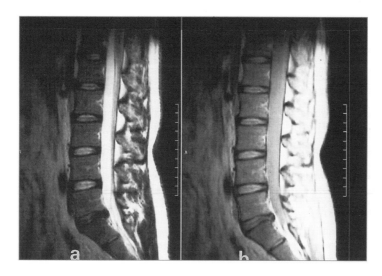

Fig. 11.33a,b. Sagittal fast spin echo images (TR 3400 ms) showing a prolapsed L5/S1 disc. **a** T2-weighted image (effective TE 105 ms) showing high signal intensity from the annulus of the normal discs and a low signal intensity from the L5/S1 disc indicating degenerative changes. **b** Proton density weighted image (effective TE 15 ms) showing the anatomical detail and the true degree of disc prolapse. (Courtesy of Siemens.)

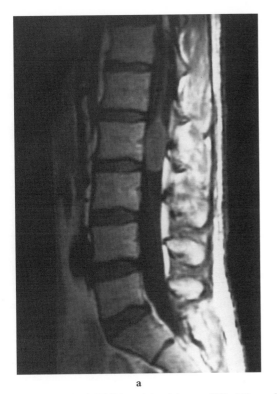 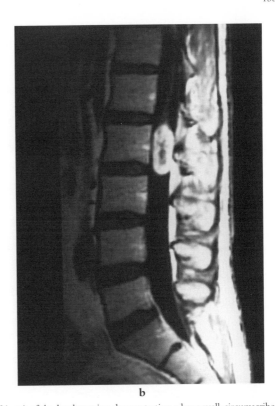

a   b

Fig. 11.34a Sagittal SE T1-weighted image (TR 450 ms, TE 21 ms) of the lumbar spine demonstrating a large well-circumscribed lesion at L2. **b** After i.v. contrast medium the lesion has enhanced and shows a necrotic centre (ependymoma of the filum).

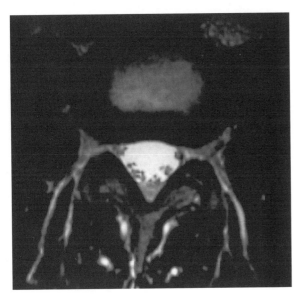 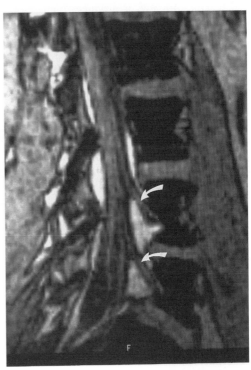

Fig. 11.35. Axial fast spin echo T2-weighted image (TR 400 ms, TE 20 ms) demonstrating the nerve roots. (Courtesy of IGE Medical Systems.)

Fig. 11.36. A reformat from a 3DFT volume acquisition showing the nerve roots (*curved arrows*) as they exit through the foramina. (Courtesy of Picker International Ltd.)

Phased array coils are now available which allow a large FOV to be covered by one acquisition. The images are of a very high quality.

3DFT volume acquisitions are also a possibility in the lumbar spine, allowing multiplanar reformats to demonstrate the nerve roots in their entirety as they exit through the foramina (Fig. 11.36).

BRACHIAL PLEXUS

The multiplanar capability of MRI together with its soft tissue contrast allow the anatomical features of the brachial plexus to be imaged in order to exclude a lesion.

Technical Considerations

Technically the brachial plexus is difficult to image because of its extent from cervical to shoulder region. A surface coil, although it produces high-resolution images, will limit the effective area scanned and only the body coil is capable of scanning such large areas. With the use of an off-centre, small FOV it is possible to obtain adequate images. In order to complete the examination further images can be obtained using a surface coil to demonstrate the spinal canal and foramina.

Patient Positioning

The patient is comfortably positioned and immobilised if possible.

Pulse Sequences

A spin echo pulse sequence is used when scanning the brachial plexus. Both T1- and T2-weighted sequences are performed.

STIR is sometimes a useful alternative to a T2-weighted sequence.

Gradient echo sequences are not usually used because of the vascular and respiratory artifacts that are generated in this region.

Scanning Planes

The coronal and axial planes are the most informative for demonstrating the anatomy of the brachial plexus. However, the brachial plexus is often examined in conjunction with the cervical spine, so the sagittal plane may also be employed.

T1-weighted coronal images are usually acquired initially. A 3–5 mm slice thickness is used with a 25–30 cm FOV and 256 reconstruction matrix.

A T2-weighted axial sequence is prescribed from C5 down to T3/4 using a 5–7 mm slice thickness, 25 cm FOV and 256 reconstruction matrix.

Contrast Enhancement

Contrast medium is not routinely used, although if a neurofibroma were suspected contrast would be beneficial.

Problem Areas

Respiration artifacts are a problem encountered in this area and can be reduced by respiratory compensation (ROPE, EXORCIST). Signal averaging will also reduce the artifact but at the expense of an increase in scanning time.

Vascular artifacts can also cause problems. The use of presaturation slabs (inferiorly) can help reduce these. Peripheral gating and gradient moment nulling can help to minimise them on the T2-weighted sequence.

Aliasing (wraparound) can be prevented by using antialiasing techniques.

New Improved Techniques

The fast spin echo sequence can reduce the scanning time of the T2-weighted sequence and thus allow a second plane to be acquired.

The advent of new vascular surface coils to image the entire length of carotid arteries from the aortic arch to the brain may also have the additional benefit of allowing high-quality surface coil images of the brachial plexus to be obtained.

HEAD AND NECK

MRI is the imaging modality of choice for many lesions of the extracranial head and neck. The ability to show the extent and infiltration of tumours and the soft tissue boundaries also helps in the planning of surgery or radiotherapy.

Technical Considerations

The head coil can be used for nasopharynx, paranasal sinuses and pharynx. A volume surface coil should be used for neck, thyroid, parathyroid glands and larynx. Alternatively anterior neck coils are available.

Patient Positioning

The patient is positioned comfortably and immobilised within the head coil or volume surface coil.

Pulse Sequences

The spin echo pulse sequence is used and T1-weighted images are obtained through the area of interest as well as a T2-weighted sequence in the most appropriate plane.

The STIR sequence can be beneficial to suppress the signal from fat and may help to reveal any underlying pathology such as enlarged lymph nodes (Fig. 11.37).

Scanning Planes

A coronal T1-weighted sequence is performed using a FOV of 25–30 mm, slice thickness of 5 mm and a 256 reconstruction matrix.

An axial T1-weighted sequence is prescribed through the area of interest using a FOV of 15–20 cm, slice thickness of 5 mm and a 256 reconstruction matrix.

Imaging in the sagittal plane may be useful to demonstrate trachea and larynx using a FOV of 25–30 cm, slice thickness of 5 mm and 256 reconstruction matrix.

The T2-weighted sequence can be performed in the most appropriate plane and/or a STIR sequence.

Contrast Enhancement

Intravenous contrast medium can be valuable in assessing the extent of a lesion. It may also have a role in assessing lymph node involvement.

Problem Areas

Swallowing and respiration cause artifacts in this region which are difficult to resolve. However, good patient cooperation together with the application of presaturation pulses and respiratory compensation will help to reduce these. Signal averaging also helps a great deal. Modern dental amalgam and the dense bone of the mandible do not degrade MR images in the way that they do CT images.

Aliasing (wraparound) can be prevented by using antialiasing techniques.

New Improved Techniques

Use of the fast spin echo sequence can minimise scanning time and in so doing help to reduce some of the motion artifacts.

MR angiography can be beneficial for demonstrating the involvement of the carotid arteries or jugular veins. The advent of vascular surface coils allows the carotid artery or jugular veins to be imaged in their entirety (Fig. 11.38).

Imaging of Different Regions of the Head and Neck

Larynx

MRI is extremely useful in delineating the stage of any disease and its extension into adjacent tissues. The high soft tissue contrast and multiplanar capabilities of MRI allow visualisation of detailed anatomy and pathology using a surface coil.

T1-weighted images are acquired in all three planes using a spin echo pulse sequence and T2-weighted images are performed in the axial plane. Relatively thin sections of 4 mm or less are used.

Oral Cavity

The most common malignant tumour of the oral cavity is squamous cell carcinoma of the tongue and floor of mouth. It is often difficult to identify as it has a low signal on T1- and T2-weighted images. Contrast administration may help. The STIR sequence will

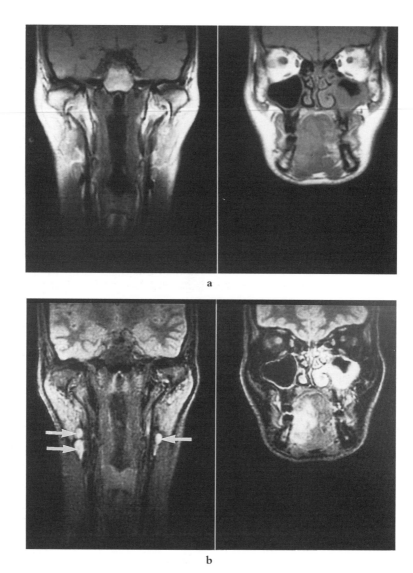

Fig. 11.37 **a** Coronal SE T1-weighted images (TR 450 ms, TE 21 ms) in the neck demonstrate anatomical detail but tissue differentiation is difficult due to the high signal from the fat. **b** Using a STIR sequence (TR 2000 ms, TI 100 ms, TE 25 ms) in the same patient suppresses the signal from fat and demonstrates enlarged lymph nodes, highly suggestive of tumour spread (*arrows*). The abnormality in the tongue (squamous cell carcinoma) is also more clearly defined.

often be helpful in delineating the extent of the lesion (Fig. 11.37).

MRI is useful for determining the full extent of the lesion as well as looking for local (lymph node) spread.

Thyroid and Parathyroid Glands

The axial plane is usually the best for delineating the normal anatomy. T1- and T2-weighted images are acquired and the STIR sequence will be beneficial for suppressing the signal from fat and detecting lesions.

Thin sections of 5 mm with a 20–25 cm FOV and a 256 matrix are required for optimal resolution, used with a surface coil.

The parathyroid glands are sometimes located within the mediastinum, and so it is important to scan into the chest when an abnormality is not present in the neck.

MUSCULOSKELETAL SYSTEM

MRI can be used very successfully in the evaluation of musculoskeletal conditions. The multiplanar facility,

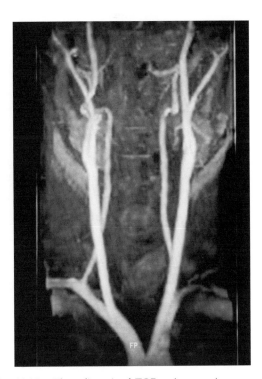

Fig. 11.38. Three-dimensional TOF angiogram using a vascular neck coil demonstrating the arterial vessels of the neck from the aortic arch up. (Courtesy of Picker International Ltd.)

the soft tissue contrast available and the ability to image changes in the bone marrow make MRI ideal in this area. The anatomical information that can be obtained when evaluating soft tissue tumours and infection is important in tumour staging and surgical planning.

Patient positioning and use of surface coils will depend on the area under investigation and the size of the patient. Imaging of the chest and abdomen will usually require a body coil, as would simultaneous imaging of both lower extremities. For small patients or children the head coil may be used. Small patients can be placed on pads to raise the area of interest as near to the isocentre of the magnet as possible. A surface coil can be used to give more detailed higher-resolution images of a single extremity. The upper extremities are more difficult to image simultaneously because of hardware limitations of the machine's maximum FOV. Therefore the upper extremities should be imaged individually using a surface coil, with the area of interest as close to the isocentre of the magnet as possible.

Imaging of Different Regions of the Musculoskeletal System

The Hip

Excellent visualisation of the soft tissue and cartilaginous structures in conjunction with small surface coils makes MRI a valuable technique for imaging the hip. Since it is extremely sensitive to changes in the marrow fat it is ideal in the assessment of avascular necrosis (AVN) and bone marrow diseases. Osteomyelitis, osteoporosis, joint effusions, Perthes disease, etc., can all be visualised using MRI, making early diagnosis possible.

Technical Considerations

When imaging both hips for comparison purposes the body coil is adequate; alternatively for greater resolution dual (butterfly) surface coils can be used. For a single hip a single circular coil or Helmholtz coil can be used.

Patient Positioning

The patient is placed supine with the legs extended and toes pointing inwards.

If surface coils are used they are positioned on the anterior pelvic wall above the appropriate hip, or suspended by some means in this position.

Pulse Sequences

The spin echo sequence is routinely used to image the hip. Multiple spin echo sequences are also used, giving proton density and T2 weighing.

STIR is useful for identifying metastatic deposits within the hip and pelvis.

Gradient echo techniques can be used to demonstrate the hyaline cartilage.

Scanning Planes

The coronal plane is used to give good anatomical detail. A T1-weighted and a multiple echo sequence are acquired in this plane. When a single hip is imaged an oblique coronal plane should be considered, allowing better visualisation of the head and neck of the femur.

When using the body coil a 35–42 cm FOV is used with a 4–5 mm slice thickness and 10% slice gap to cover the whole hip joint. A 256 reconstruction matrix is used for high-resolution images. When using a surface coil resolution can be further improved by reducing the FOV to 20 cm.

T1-weighted images are also acquired in the axial plane, with similar parameters according to coil type. Oblique axial images can sometimes be useful when imaging femoral neck pathology.

Sagittal images of the affected hip are sometimes acquired but not routinely.

AVN is one of the most commonly encountered pathologies in the hip, as shown in Fig. 11.39.

Contrast Enhancement

Intravenous contrast medium is not routinely used in the hip joint, although MR arthrography is currently under evaluation.

Problem areas

Vascular artifacts can sometimes obscure the joint, especially on axial images. Presaturation pulses (superiorly and inferiorly) help minimise these. Gradient moment nulling for the multiple echo sequence also helps.

New Improved Techniques

The fast spin echo sequence will allow short acquisition times for a T2-weighted sequence. Three-dimensional volume acquisitions may improve resolution of hip pathologies.

The Knee

MRI is excellent for evaluating the knee for internal derangement and in many cases has replaced arthrography. It is particularly useful for meniscal and ligamentous injuries. The protocol used will depend upon the capabilities of the imaging system employed.

Technical Considerations

Most imagers have dedicated knee coils which are often the transmit/receive type. Other types include wraparound coils, loop-gap resonator coils and saddle-shaped coils.

Patient Positioning

The patient is positioned supine, feet first, with the affected knee in the coil so that the centre of the joint is at the centre of the coil. The leg is relaxed and this results in approximately 10°–15° of external rotation – a position that allows easy visualisation of the anterior cruciate ligament. Sponges should be used to stabilise the leg in this position.

Pulse Sequences

The spin echo sequence is used to acquire T1-weighted images along with a multiple spin echo sequence to give proton density and T2-weighted information.

A gradient echo sequence can also be used. If the parameters are set correctly it is possible to distinguish between joint fluid and hyaline cartilage.

STIR sequences are useful in cases of tumour to define the extent of the lesion more accurately, and in cases of trauma to evaluate the degree of bone bruising.

Scanning Planes

The sagittal plane is useful for the demonstration of the cruciate ligaments, menisci, femoropatellar, joint and cartilaginous lesions.

Coronal and axial images must also be acquired to complete the examination, or lesions such as bucket-handle tears and collateral ligament ruptures could be missed. Meniscal cysts are easily identified on a coronal sequence. The axial image is valuable for showing the femoropatellar articular surface in suspected disorders. Axial images of the menisci require double oblique planes but can sometimes show the intermeniscal ligament in its entirety.

T1-, proton density and T2-weighted sequences are acquired in the sagittal plane using a 15–20 cm FOV, a slice thickness of 3–4 mm with a 10% slice gap, and a 256 reconstruction matrix. An interleaving technique can be used which allows the acquisition of contiguous or overlapping slices without "cross-talk" between the slices (Fig. 11.40).

There are various methods of ensuring that the sagittal slices are angled correctly to show the anterior cruciate ligament. In our experience angling to the lateral border of the lateral femoral condyle will demonstrate it well (see Fig. 11.40). Another technique is the use of a template which allows the slices to be prescribed in respect of the posterior femoral condyles.

The sagittal images should cover from the outer aspect of one femoral condyle to the outer aspect of the other.

T1-weighted images are also acquired in the coronal and axial planes using a 15–20 cm FOV, a slice thickness of 3–4 mm and a 256 reconstruction matrix. The axial images should cover the knee from the tibial tuberosity to the suprapatellar region. The coronal images should be angled to the posterior margins of the femoral condyles using the appropriate axial image, covering from the posterior femoral condyles to the patella.

When assessing meniscal abnormalities it can be useful to image the appropriate sagittal and coronal slices both with conventional settings and using a narrow window width to produce high-contrast images which are zoomed to the meniscus.

Contrast Enhancement

Contrast enhancement is not routinely used in the knee joint. A recent study suggests greater conspicuity of meniscal tears after i.v. contrast medium. MR arthrography can be of value in difficult cases of loose bodies.

Problem Areas

Vascular flow artifacts from the popliteal vessels can substantially degrade the central sagittal images. Swapping the phase-encoding axis from the Y (anteroposterior) to the Z (head to foot) direction places the artifacts away from the area of most interest. Presaturation slabs help to minimise the artifacts. Gradient moment nulling can be used in the multiple echo sequence to reduce the artifacts further.

Aliasing (wraparound) can occur when using a small FOV. Antialiasing techniques will remove the artifact from the image.

Pathology and Pitfalls

The menisci of the knee are composed of fibrocartilage and are normally demonstrated as wedge-shaped

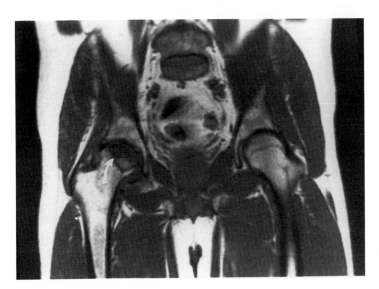

Fig. 11.39. Coronal SE T1-weighted image (TR 450 ms, TE 21 ms) of the hips showing an abnormal low signal area within one femoral head (*arrow*) caused by avascular necrosis.

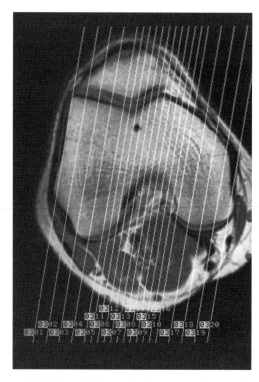

Fig. 11.40. Axial SE T1-weighted image (TR 450 ms, TE 21 ms) showing the interleaving technique, with the slices angled to the lateral femoral condyle in order to demonstrate the anterior cruciate ligament.

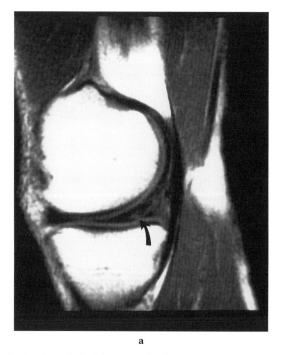

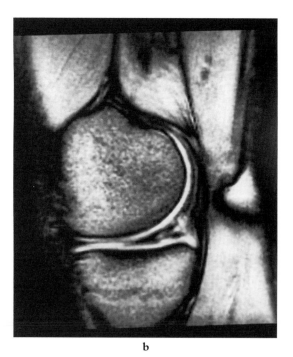

a   b

Fig. 11.41 **a** Sagittal SE T1-weighted image (TR 450 ms, TE 21 ms) of the knee demonstrating a tear of the posterior horn of the medial meniscus (*arrow*). **b** Sagittal T2* gradient echo image (TR 400 ms, TE 21 ms, flip angle 45°) demonstrating the same tear but more clearly as a result of the different contrast generated by the sequence.

hyperintense structures in all pulse sequences. The menisci are seen as "bow–tie" structures on peripheral sections in the sagittal plane, whilst more central sections show the separate anterior and posterior horns of the menisci.

A discoid meniscus is suspected if the meniscus remains solid on more than two slices of 5 mm thickness. This can be confirmed on the coronal sequence as the abnormal meniscus often extends to or into the intercondylar notch. The easiest way of distinguishing from which side a section originates is either by the characteristic shape of the tibial plateau (which is concave medially and convex laterally) or by visualising the fibula (which is on the lateral aspect of the leg). Occasionally a normal meniscus displays an internal band of intermediate or high signal which follows the meniscal contour. This does not represent a tear and the reason for this signal is not fully understood. It is only if the signal extends from the inner substance of the meniscus to its surface that a tear is diagnosed (Fig. 11.41). The high signal intensity associated with a torn meniscus results from the synovial fluid which diffuses through the meniscus. The other indication of a meniscal tear is a change in the size and shape of a meniscus. Tears may be classified as radial, vertical, parrot's beak, bucket handle or displaced fragments, and are graded into four categories.

The popliteal tendon is seen as an area of low signal intensity as it courses obliquely posterior to the lateral meniscus, and the tendon sheath can sometimes mimic a tear of the posterior horn.

The anterior cruciate ligament (ACL) is a band-like structure, often showing striations, that extends obliquely (about 15° from the sagittal plane) and is inserted at the internal aspect of the lateral femoral condyle to the anterior aspect of the tibial spine. The ACL protects the knee from hyperextension and is the knee ligament that is most frequently torn. It has a slightly different signal characteristic from the posterior cruciate ligament. When the knee is extended the ACL is straight. Total ACL disruption (Fig. 11.42) is evidenced by disruption along the normal smooth course, or by failure to demonstrate the ligament on a series of contiguous or interleaved thin slices. Partial tears are diagnosed when the integrity of the ligament is preserved but there are areas of increased signal intensity within it (Fig. 11.42). A useful sign of an ACL tear is an abnormal shape to the posterior cruciate ligament, which looks straighter and has a hook-shaped appearance near the femoral attachment.

The posterior cruciate ligament (PCL) is a smooth curved band extending from the internal aspect of the medial condyle to the posterior aspect of the tibia. It stabilises the medial femoral condyle during flexion and prevents backward displacement of the tibia on the femur. It is curved when the knee is in extension. The anterior and posterior meniscofemoral ligaments (ligaments of Humphry and Wrisberg) are closely related to the PCL and may simulate a tear of the posterior horn of the meniscus. The ligament of Humphry produces a localised anterior thickening of the PCL and may be separate from the PCL, and thus be confused with an intra-articular loose body. Disruption of the PCL is demonstrated as loss of ligament continuity.

The medial and lateral collateral ligaments are best visualised on coronal images but can also be seen on axial images as bands of uniformly low signal. A tear of a collateral ligament reveals abnormal signal intensity and disruption of the smooth course of the ligament. Oedema, blood or fluid at the site of injury, increased thickness and discontinuity of the ligament may be well demonstrated on T2-weighted sequences as a high signal intensity.

Fluid collections in the knee are easily visualised on T1-weighted sequences and T2-weighted sequences are not usually required.

MRI can also help to diagnose other abnormalities such as osteochondritis dissecans (Fig. 11.43) before plain radiographs are abnormal. Following trauma it is possible to demonstrate abnormalities in the soft tissues surrounding the knee, such as quadriceps tendon tears or ruptures, popliteal cysts and intramuscular haematomas. Chondromalacia patellae is an important cause of knee pain and MRI is sensitive to the thinning and degenerative change of the hyaline cartilage.

New Improved Techniques

Magnetisation transfer has been used in the knee, allowing better differentiation between the hyaline cartilage and the synovial fluid. Improvements in surface coil design and the development of phased array coils will further improve resolution.

A 512 reconstruction matrix in the knee allows extremely high-resolution images to be acquired, and combining this technique with fast spin echo sequences improves resolution even further (Fig. 11.44).

Three-dimensional volume acquisitions allow retrospective multiplanar reformats of the knee, which enables the entire knee to be examined with just one sequence (Fig. 11.45).

Kinematic imaging of the knee is performed in the axial plane to assess patellar instability. This is achieved by scanning in the prone position and performing repeated scans at the same location, starting with the knee extended and gradually flexing it, with scans repeated every 5° of flexion. Once acquired the images can be played back in a cine loop.

Radial scanning is a technique which allows multiple oblique sections to be acquired in a radial fashion. This enables images to be obtained directly perpendicular to the meniscus and is achieved by rapid gradient switching (Fig. 11.46).

The Ankle/Foot

MRI has proved useful in the evaluation of many abnormalities of the ankle and foot. Avascular necrosis, tendon lesions/ruptures/entrapment, ligament tears, Achilles tendon rupture, joint effusions, infections and osteochondral lesions can all be visualised on MRI.

Osteomyelitis can be detected by MRI in its early stages when plain radiographs are normal.

Technical Considerations

The dedicated knee coil, which is usually of the transmit/receive type, can be used to image the ankle. Other types include wraparound coils, loop-gap resonator coils and saddle-shaped coils.

The tarsal bones can be imaged using the knee coil; the forefoot, however, requires a surface coil of a different design. Solenoid coils perpendicular to the main magnetic field are used with the foot placed within them, or a linear coil with the dorsum of the foot planted firmly on the coil.

Patient Positioning

The patient is placed supine with the affected ankle or foot in the surface coil. The leg is secured as comfortably as possible.

Pulse Sequences

A T1-weighted spin echo pulse sequence is acquired preceded by a multiple spin echo sequence to give proton density and T2-weighted information.

A gradient echo sequence can also be used. If the parameters are set correctly this enables joint fluid and hyaline cartilage to be distinguished.

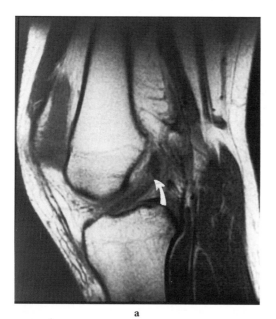

a

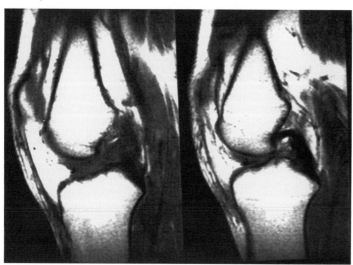

b

Fig. 11.42 a Sagittal SE T1-weighted image (TR 450 ms, TE 21 ms) of the knee demonstrating an area of intermediate signal within the anterior cruciate ligament (*arrow*) representing a partial tear. **b** Sagittal SE T1-weighted images (TR 450 ms, TE 21 ms) of the knee demonstrating a complete tear of the anterior cruciate ligament together with the characteristic "hooking" of the posterior cruciate ligament.

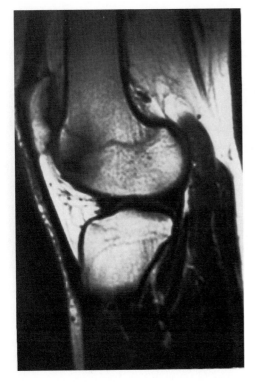

Fig. 11.43. Sagittal SE T1-weighted image (TR 450 ms, TE 21 ms) of the knee. There is an area of low signal in the femoral condyle diagnosed as osteochondritis dissecans.

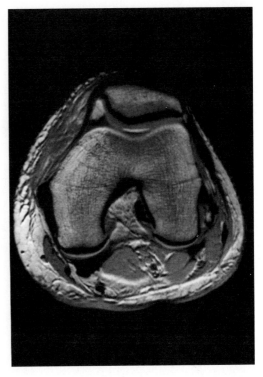

Fig. 11.44. Axial fast spin echo T1-weighted image (TR 600 ms, effective TE 30 ms) of the knee using a 512 reconstruction matrix. (Courtesy of IGE Medical Systems.)

STIR sequences are useful in cases of tumour to define the extent of the lesion more accurately, and in cases of trauma to evaluate the degree of bone bruising.

Scanning Planes

A T1-weighted spin echo pulse sequence in the axial plane is acquired using a FOV of 12–15 cm, a slice thickness of 3–5 mm and 256 reconstruction matrix.

From the appropriate axial image a coronal T1-weighted spin echo pulse sequence is performed, angling the slices between the medial and lateral malleoli. A FOV of 12–15 cm with a slice thickness of 3–5 mm and 256 reconstruction matrix are used.

A sagittal T1-weighted spin echo pulse sequence is acquired using a FOV of 12–15 cm, slice thickness of 3–5 mm and 256 reconstruction matrix.

A multiple echo sequence is performed in the most appropriate plane to give proton density and T2-weighted information. Fig. 11.47 shows the appearance of a Brodie's abscess, which is typically an isointense area on a T1-weighted sequence and hyperintense on a T2-weighted sequence.

Achilles tendon injuries require sagittal and axial images covering the area from the calcaneal insertion to the origin in the mid calf. Axial images are probably the most informative, showing any signal abnormality within the tendon consistent with a tear (Fig. 11.48). Sagittal images in plantar flexion and dorsiflexion are useful for the evaluation of Achilles tendon ruptures. These positions can also be useful in evaluating ankle ligaments.

The forefoot requires slightly different scanning planes, but using similar parameters to the ankle with a slightly larger FOV (20–25 cm) for the sagittal and axial planes. Oblique axial planes are prescribed parallel to the long axes of the metatarsal bones, oblique coronal planes perpendicular to the metatarsals, and oblique sagittal planes down the long axis of the metatarsals.

Contrast Enhancement

Contrast medium is not routinely used when imaging the ankle or foot.

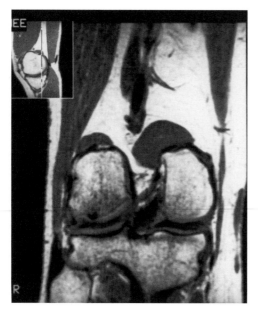

Fig. 11.45. Coronal reformatted image of the knee from a sagittal 3DFT T1-weighted gradient echo series. (TR 30 ms, TE 13 ms, flip angle 45°). (Courtesy of Philips Medical Systems.)

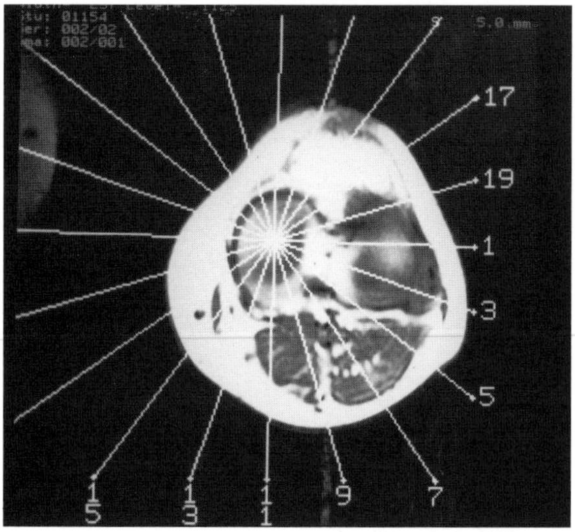

Fig. 11.46. Radial imaging of the meniscus. An axial image from a 3DFT volume set is used to prescribe planes for reconstructing radial images of the meniscus. (Courtesy of IGE Medical Systems.)

Problem Areas

The use of a small FOV can cause aliasing in the sagittal images. This can be prevented by using an antialiasing technique.

New Improved Techniques

Improvements in surface coil design and the use of phased array coils will further improve resolution.

A 512 reconstruction matrix in the ankle/foot allows highly resolved images to be acquired and combining this technique with fast spin echo sequences gives the ability to obtain very high-resolution T2-weighted images.

Three-dimensional volume acquisitions allow multiplanar reconstruction of the ankle/foot allowing the entire ankle/foot to be examined with just one sequence.

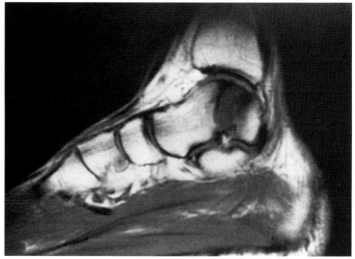

Fig. 11.47 a,b. Sagittal and coronal SE T1-weighted images respectively (TR 450 ms, TE 21 ms) of the ankle showing a hypointense area in the talus. **c** Coronal SE T2-weighted images (TR 2000 ms, TE 80 ms) in the same patient showing a hyperintense area with a hypointense rim representing a dense fibrous capsule or sclerotic reactive bone. This was diagnosed as a Brodie's abscess.

a

Fig. 11.48. Axial SE T2-weighted image (TR 2000 ms, TE 80 ms) of the ankle demonstrating an abnormal area of intermediate signal intensity within the Achilles tendon (*arrow*). Anteriorly there is a large haemorrhagic collection associated with the abnormality. These are post-traumatic changes in a patient with an incomplete rupture of the Achilles tendon.

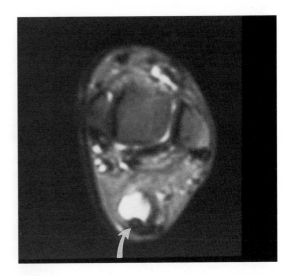

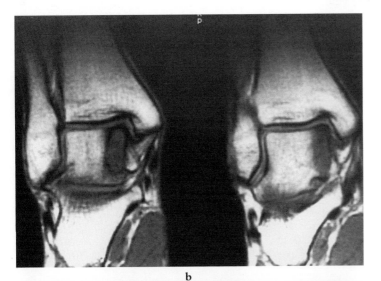

b

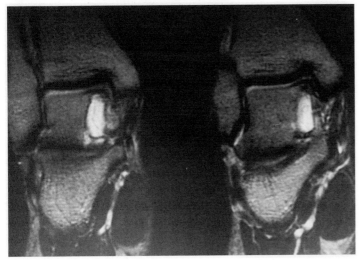

c

The Shoulder

MRI is proving to be equal, if not superior, to other available imaging modalities in the evaluation of shoulder problems including impingement syndrome, osteonecrosis of the humeral head, glenohumeral instability, tendonitis of the supraspinatus tendon, rotator cuff tears (Fig, 11.49), synovial lesions, bursitis and avascular necrosis.

Technical Considerations

There are a number of coils available for imaging the shoulder joint, including dedicated linear, quadrature, loop-gap, flexible wraparound and Helmholtz coils.

Patient Positioning

The patient is placed supine, head first into the scanner. The arm is placed by the side and externally rotated.

Pulse Sequences

Spin echo T1-weighted pulse sequences are acquired together with a multiple echo sequence to give proton density and T2-weighted information.

A gradient echo sequence can also be used. If the parameters are set correctly this enables joint fluid and hyaline cartilage to be distinguished.

STIR sequences are useful in cases of tumour to define the extent of the lesion more accurately and in cases of trauma to evaluate the degree of bone bruising.

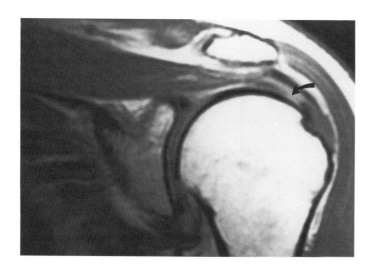

Fig. 11.49. Coronal SE T1-weighted image (TR 450 ms, TE 21 ms) of the shoulder showing an area of hyperintensity (*arrow*) in the region of the supraspinatus tendon representing a tear of the rotator cuff.

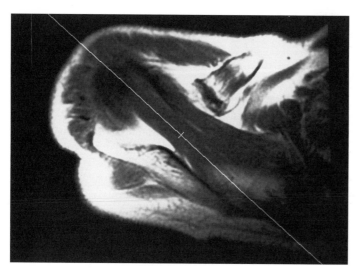

Fig. 11.50. Axial SE T1-weighted image (TR 450 ms, TE 21 ms) of the shoulder demonstrating the angle along the long axis of the supraspinatus muscle used to prescribe the oblique coronal images.

Scanning Planes

For a complete examination of the shoulder joint scans in all three orthogonal planes should be performed.

A T1-weighted sequence in the oblique coronal plane prescribed from an appropriate axial image, angling along the length of the supraspinatus muscle (Fig. 11.50), is acquired to demonstrate the muscles and tendon of the rotator cuff, the subacromial region and the acromioclavicular joint.

A multiple echo sequence can also be performed in this plane to give proton density and T2-weighted information. A FOV of 15–20 cm, slice thickness of 3–5 mm and 256 reconstruction matrix can be used.

The axial plane demonstrates the glenoid labrum, biceps tendon, subscapularis tendon and the bicipital groove, and is prescribed from an appropriate coronal image. A T2-weighted sequence in the axial plane is useful if labral tear or capsular detachment is suspected. A FOV of 15–20 cm, slice thickness of 3–5 mm and 256 reconstruction matrix are used.

Sagittal oblique planes prescribed along the transverse axis of the supraspinatus muscle will also demonstrate the muscles and tendons of the rotator cuff as well as the anatomy of the acromioclavicular arch and the subacromial structures. A FOV of 15–20 cm, slice thickness of 3–5 mm and 256 reconstruction matrix are used.

When imaging both shoulders for avascular necrosis, the body coil can be used to image them simultaneously.

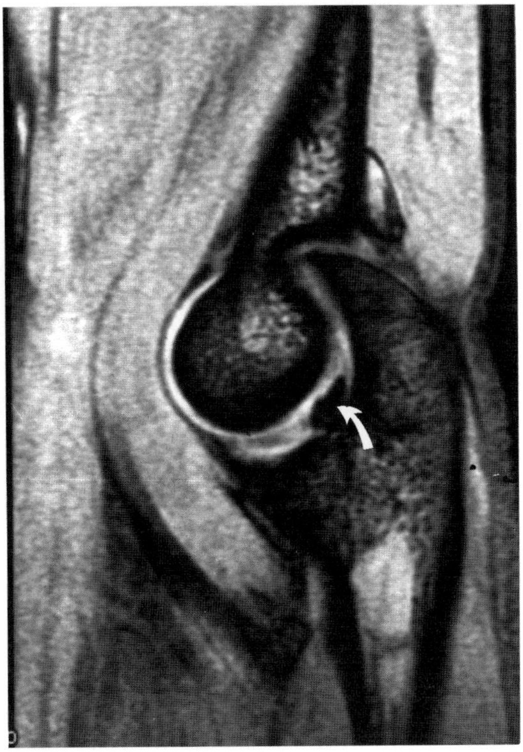

Contrast Enhancement

Contrast medium is not routinely used. Shoulder arthrograms can sometimes be performed to give better detail of the intracapsular structures.

Problem Areas

Respiratory motion can cause artifacts which will degrade the images. These can be reduced by using respiratory compensation or signal averaging.

The use of a small FOV can cause wraparound (aliasing). This can be prevented by using an antialiasing technique.

New Improved Techniques

Improvements in surface coil design and the development of phased array coils will further improve resolution.

A 512 reconstruction matrix in the shoulder allows extremely highly resolved images to be acquired and combining this technique with the fast spin echo sequence gives the ability to obtain very high-resolution T2-weighted images.

Three-dimensional volume acquisitions allow multiplanar reconstruction of the shoulder which enables the entire shoulder to be examined with just one sequence.

The Elbow

MRI can provide useful information, particularly in soft tissue lesions but also to demonstrate synovial cysts, joint effusion, osteochondral lesions, loose bodies (Fig. 11.51) and osteochondritis dissecans (which is frequently related to sports trauma).

Technical Considerations

The elbow can be examined using a general-purpose receive-only linear coil, a wraparound coil or other suitable extremity coil, depending on what is available.

Fig. 11.51. Sagittal three-dimensional gradient echo sequence (TR 47 ms, TE 11 ms) of the elbow joint demonstrating a loose body (*arrow*) in the joint space. (Courtesy of IGE Medical Systems.)

Patient Positioning

The elbow can be scanned in one of two positions: with the arm above the head (but this is an extremely uncomfortable position to maintain for any length of time) or, preferably, with the arm down at the side and externally rotated with the coil placed in close proximity to the elbow. A foam pad is used to raise the elbow to the centre of the Y-axis of the magnet.

Pulse Sequences

Spin echo T1-weighted pulse sequences are acquired along with a multiple echo sequence to give proton density and T2-weighted information.

A T2★ gradient echo sequence can be valuable to demonstrate articular cartilage.

STIR sequences are useful in cases of tumour to define the extent of the lesion more accurately, and in cases of trauma to evaluate the degree of bone bruising.

Scanning Planes

T1-weighted spin echo images are acquired first in the coronal plane, followed by the sagittal plane to demonstrate the trochlear–ulnar and capitular–radial head articulations. A FOV of 15–20 cm, slice thickness of 3–5 mm and 256 reconstruction matrix will give high spatial resolution.

The axial plane will demonstrate the proximal radio-ulnar joint and T1-, proton density and T2-weighted images are acquired in this plane. A FOV of 12–15 cm, slice thickness of 3–5 mm and 256 reconstruction matrix are used.

Contrast Enhancement

Contrast medium is not routinely used.

Problem Areas

The use of a small FOV can cause wraparound (aliasing). This can be prevented by using an antialiasing technique.

Patient comfort can be a problem when imaging the elbow and some patients may have great difficulty straightening the elbow at all. In such cases imaging perpendicular to both the humerus and forearm with separate acquisitions is the only solution.

Presaturation applied above and below the imaging plane reduces vascular artifacts.

New Improved Techniques

Improvements in surface coil design and the development of phased array coils will further improve resolution.

A 512 reconstruction matrix in the elbow allows extremely highly resolved images to be acquired and combining this technique with the fast spin echo sequence gives the ability to obtain very high-resolution T2-weighted images.

Three-dimensional volume acquisitions allow multiplanar reconstruction of the elbow which enables the entire elbow to be examined with just one sequence.

The Hand and Wrist

MRI of the hand and wrist allows excellent visualisation of the wrist ligaments without using invasive techniques, as well as demonstrating compression neuropathies (carpal tunnel syndrome, Guyon's canal syndrome), neurovascular structures, ligament and tendon injuries, tenosynovitis, entrapment syndromes, ganglion cysts and avascular necrosis (Fig. 11.52).

Technical Considerations

It is essential to use a surface coil in order to obtain the high resolution required to demonstrate the anatomy of the hand and wrist. A Helmholtz or two circular receive-only coils placed above and below the hand or wrist can be used. Dedicated transmit/receive coils or wraparound coils are available for the wrist.

Patient Positioning

The patient is positioned supine, head first into the scanner, with the hand or wrist down at their side within the surface coil. A foam pad is used to raise the wrist/hand to the isocentre of the magnet and the area to be scanned is immobilised. Patients who cannot be placed supine are placed prone with the arm overhead (swimmer's position) and made as comfortable as possible. This position may be difficult to maintain for long periods of time.

Pulse Sequences

The spin echo sequence is used to acquired T1-weighted images, together with a multiple spin echo sequence to give proton density and T2-weighted information.

A gradient echo sequence can also be used. If the parameters are set correctly joint fluid and hyaline cartilage can be distinguished.

STIR sequences are useful in cases of tumour to define the extent of the lesion more accurately, and in cases of trauma to evaluate the degree of bone bruising.

Scanning Planes

T1-weighted spin echo sequences are acquired in all three anatomical planes with a multiple echo sequence acquired in the most suitable plane (usually axial). The axial plane demonstrates the anatomy of the carpal tunnel delineating tendons, ligaments, bones, muscles and neurovascular bundles. The coronal plane demonstrates the course of the tendons, nerves and blood vessels, and also shows the articular cartilage of the wrist and various ligaments. The sagittal plane best demonstrates the anatomy of the fingers.

A 3–5 mm slice thickness is used with a 10% slice gap; an 8–12 cm FOV with a 256 reconstruction matrix will suffice in all planes.

Oblique sagittal images of the individual fingers will reduce partial volume effects.

Contrast Enhancement

Contrast medium is not routinely used.

Problem Areas

The use of a small FOV can cause wraparound (aliasing) from other parts of the body. This can be prevented by using an antialiasing technique.

Presaturation applied above and below the imaging plane reduces vascular artifacts, although they are not a major problem in the wrist.

New Improved Techniques

Improvements in surface coil design and the development of phased array coils will further improve resolution.

A 512 reconstruction matrix in the hand and wrist allows extremely highly resolved images to be acquired and combining this technique with the fast spin echo sequence gives the ability to obtain very high-resolution T2-weighted images.

Three-dimensional volume acquisitions allow multiplanar reconstruction of the hand and wrist which enables the entire region of interest to be examined with just one sequence.

Kinematic imaging of the wrist is performed in the coronal plane to assess carpal instability. Once acquired the images can be played back in a cine loop.

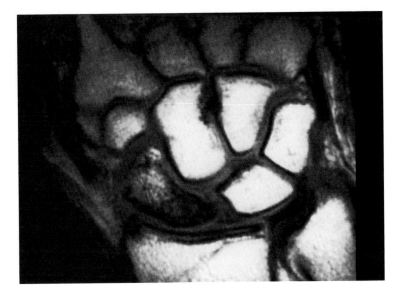

Fig. 11.52. Coronal SE T1-weighted image (TR 450 ms, TE 21 ms) of the wrist using a dedicated surface coil demonstrating avascular necrosis of the scaphoid. (Courtesy of IGE Medical Systems.)

The Temporo-mandibular Joint

Arthrography, though the investigation of choice for years when imaging the temporo-mandibular joint (TMJ), is invasive and uncomfortable for the patient. MRI has revolutionised investigation of the TMJ, its soft tissue contrast and ability to visualise the disc without the administration of contrast medium making it ideal for evaluating diseases of this joint.

Technical Considerations

A small circular 3 inch coil is used to image the TMJ. Bilateral TMJ coils are available and these allow simultaneous imaging of both joints for comparison.

Patient Positioning

The patient is place supine, head first in the scanner, with the coil or coils positioned as close to the TMJ as possible. Clear instructions need to be given to the patient regarding what is expected of them during the examination, as images are acquired with the mouth open and closed.

Pulse Sequences

T1-weighted spin echo pulse sequences are routinely used. T2-weighted images are not usually of any benefit.

Gradient echo sequences are used for kinematic studies, giving good contrast between the articular cartilage and the soft tissue structures around the joint.

Scanning Planes

The axial plane is useful for localising the TMJ and determining the degree of obliquity for the sagittal images.

The sagittal plane is ideal for imaging the TMJ; angling the slices perpendicular to the condyles of the joint achieves the best results. A 10–15 cm FOV is used together with a slice thickness of 2–3 mm and a 256 reconstruction matrix. The sagittal sequence is acquired with the mouth closed and open.

A coronal sequence, with the mouth closed, is acquired to assess medial or lateral displacement of the articular disc.

Kinematic imaging of the TMJ is performed in the sagittal plane to demonstrate mechanical functional abnormalities. A special positioning device allows the mouth to be opened gradually by predetermined increments, a scan being acquired in each position. Once acquired the images can be played back in a cine loop.

Contrast Enhancement

Contrast medium is not routinely used.

Problem Areas

The use of a small FOV can cause wraparound (aliasing) in the sagittal images. This can be prevented by using an antialiasing technique.

New Improved Techniques

Improvements in surface coil design and the development of quadrature coils will further improve resolution.

A 512 reconstruction matrix in the TMJ allows extremely highly resolved images to be acquired and combining this technique with a fast spin echo sequence gives the ability to obtain very high-resolution T2-weighted images.

LONG BONES

The type of coil used for the long bones will depend upon the area of interest to be covered. A surface coil should be used if the area of interest can be localised, as this will give better contrast and resolution.

Common Parameters Used when Imaging the Long Bones

Pulse Sequences

The spin echo sequence is used and both T1- and T2-weighted images are acquired.

STIR sequences can be useful in cases of tumour to define the extent of the lesion more accurately, and in lipomatous lesions (Fig. 11.53) and cases of trauma to evaluate the degree of bone bruising.

Gradient echo sequences are useful in evaluating soft tissues as well as for reducing acquisition times and allowing thin slices to be used. Axial gradient echo

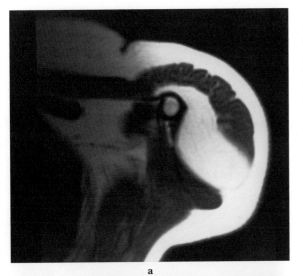

a

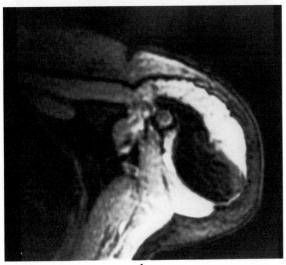

b

Fig. 11.53. a Axial SE T1-weighted image (TR 500 ms, TE 21 ms) of the proximal humerus demonstrating an abnormal area of hyperintensity in the region of the deltoid. **b** Axial STIR image (TR 2000 ms, TI 100 ms, TE 25 ms) has suppressed the signal from the lesion as well as the subcutaneous fat. These are the MRI appearances of a lipoma.

sequences can be used to highlight blood vessels and show their proximity to lesions.

Scanning Planes

Images in three orthogonal planes may be required to complete the examination, with T2-weighted and/or STIR sequences being acquired in the most appropriate plane.

A sagittal or coronal localiser is acquired using a FOV large enough to demonstrate the extent of abnormality. Axial or coronal slices are prescribed from this using a FOV large enough to cover the area of interest, a slice thickness of 5–10 mm and a 256 reconstruction matrix. The exact selection of parameters depends upon the sensitivity of the coil being used. The FOV and matrix selection will vary according to the scanning plane and coverage required.

When imaging the long bones it is useful to obtain oblique planes along the longitudinal axis of the bone, especially in cases of tumour as this will show the intra- and extraosseous extent of the tumour (Fig. 11.54) and its relationship to surrounding structures in one slice.

The sagittal plane is sometimes beneficial when assessing marrow changes.

Imaging of the Different Long Bones

Femur

Technical Considerations

If the full extent of the femur is to be imaged or if scans of femora are required for comparison purposes, then the body coil can be used. An appropriate surface coil can be used for localised areas.

Patient Positioning

The patient is placed supine with the legs extended and the toes pointing inwards and made as comfortable as possible.

Scanning Planes and Pulse Sequences

The spin echo pulse sequence is used and both T1- and T2-weighted images are acquired.

The coronal and axial planes allow direct comparison of right and left femora (Fig. 11.55).

A FOV of 40–50 cm will usually cover both femora using a 256 matrix. A slice thickness of 5–10 mm is used, depending upon the clinical indications.

Contrast Enhancement

Contrast medium is not routinely used although it can provide additional information in certain cases.

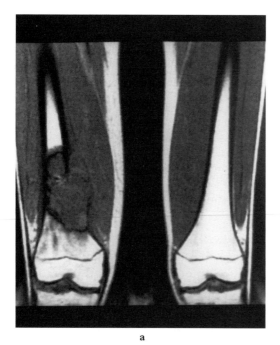
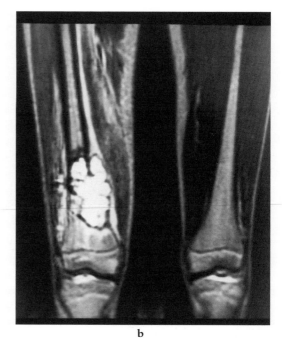

a   b

Fig. 11.54 a Coronal SE T1-weighted image (TR 500 ms, TE 21 ms) of the distal femur showing a hypointense area which appears to extend both intraosseously and extraosseously. **b** Coronal SE T2-weighted image (TR 2000 ms, TE 80 ms) of the femur allows the extent of the lesion to be more clearly delineated (osteosarcoma).

Problem Areas

Vascular artifacts can be reduced by the application of presaturation pulses placed superiorly and inferiorly.

New Improved Techniques

Fast spin echo techniques allow T2-weighted sequences to be acquired in multiple planes.

Peripheral MR angiography of the femoral vessels can be used to evaluate vascular problems.

Tibia and Fibula

Technical Considerations

In certain instances the body coil (or the head coil, if the patient is small enough) may be used to cover the whole leg and for direct comparison of right and left legs. More commonly a surface coil is employed to give high-definition images.

Patient Positioning

The patient is placed supine, feet first into the scanner.

The leg is extended and immobilised in a comfortable position, ensuring that the area of interest is within the sensitive range of the coil selected.

Pulse Sequences and Scanning Planes

The spin echo pulse sequence is used and both T1- and T2-weighted images are acquired in the appropriate planes (Fig. 11.56).

A large FOV (30–45 cm) when using the body coil will give adequate coverage of both legs for comparison. The large FOV also allows full coverage in the coronal and sagittal planes of any involved muscles and associated tendons. When using a surface coil a FOV of 25–35 cm, 5–10 mm slice thickness and 256 reconstruction matrix will give high-resolution images.

Contrast Enhancement

Contrast medium is not routinely used although can provide additional information in certain cases.

Problem Areas

Vascular artifacts can be reduced by the application of presaturation pulses placed superiorly and inferiorly.

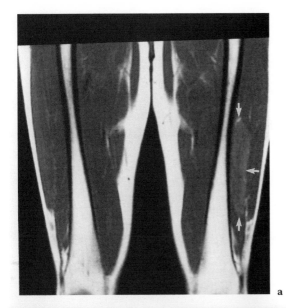

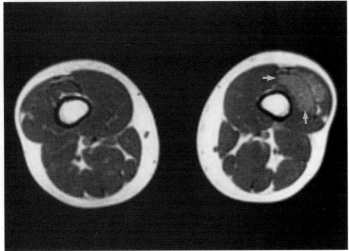

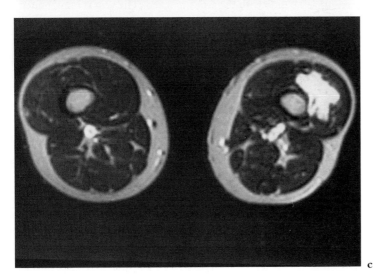

Fig. 11.55 a Coronal SE T1-weighted image (TR 500 ms, TE 21 ms) of the distal femur showing an area that is hyperintense (*arrow*) compared with the surrounding muscle. **b** Axial SE T1-weighted image (TR 500 ms, TE 21 ms) showing the lesion extending into the vastus intermedius muscle (*arrows*). **c** Axial SE T2-weighted image (TR 2000 ms, TE 80 ms) showing the lesion to be hyperintense. No abnormality is demonstrated in the bone. This was found to be an intramuscular haemangioma.

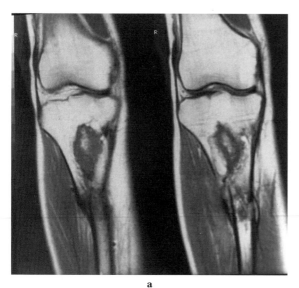

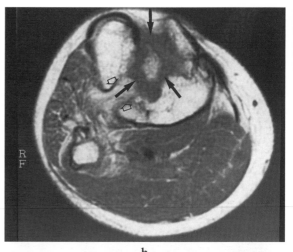

b

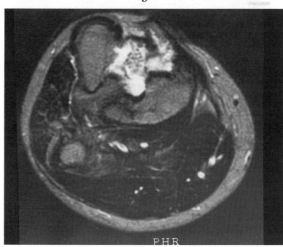

c

Fig. 11.56 **a** Coronal SE T1-weighted image (TR 500 ms, TE 21 ms) of the proximal tibia in a patient with an old fracture showing an area of hypointensity within the bone. **b** Axial SE T1-weighted image (TR 500 ms, TE 21 ms) showing the old un-united fracture (*open arrows*) and an abnormal signal around the fracture site (*filled arrows*). **c** Axial SE T2-weighted image (TR 2000 ms, TE 80 ms) showing this area to be hyperintense. This was found to be osteomyelitis.

New Improved Techniques

Fast spin echo techniques allow T2-weighted sequences to be acquired in multiple planes.

Peripheral MR angiography can be used to evaluate vascular problems.

Humerus

Technical Considerations

The body coil can be used to enable the whole of the humerus to be imaged; alternatively a rectangular coil could be used. An appropriate surface coil can be used for localised areas.

Patient Positioning

The patient is placed supine, head first into the scan-

ner. In order to achieve the true anatomical position the patient could be rotated slightly onto the affected side with the arm supinated. The arm is immobilised in a comfortable position, ensuring that the area of interest is within the sensitive range of the coil selected.

Pulse Sequences and Scanning Planes

The spin echo pulse sequence is used and both T1- and T2-weighted images are acquired.

To cover the entire humerus in the coronal or sagittal plane a large FOV of 35–45 cm is required together with a 5–7 mm slice thickness and a 256 reconstruction matrix.

Contrast Enhancement

Contrast medium is not routinely used although it can provide extra information in certain cases.

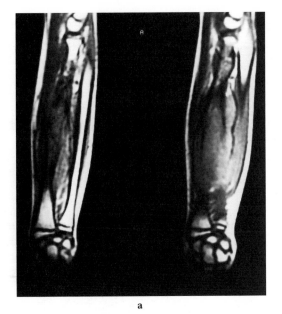
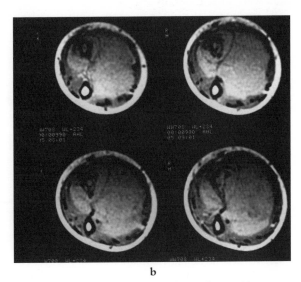

Fig. 11.57 **a** Coronal SE T1-weighted image (TR 450 ms, TE 21 ms) of the forearm showing a large soft tissue lesion with apparent destruction of the mid-shaft of the radius. **b** Axial SE T1-weighted image (TR 500 ms, TE 21 ms) shows the full extent of the surrounding soft tissue involvement and also how the ulna is left apparently unaffected (osteosarcoma).

Problem Areas

Vascular artifacts can be reduced by the application of presaturation pulses placed superiorly and inferiorly. Cardiac and respiratory motion cause problems when the phase-encoding axis is in the *Y*-axis (left to right); a presaturation slab placed to cover the chest will reduce these artifacts.

Wraparound (aliasing) can occur from the chest when a small FOV is employed. An antialiasing technique will minimise these artifacts.

New Improved Techniques

Fast spin echo techniques allow T2-weighted sequences to be acquired in multiple planes.

Radius and Ulna

Technical Considerations

A rectangular surface coil can be used to cover the whole length of the radius and ulna.

Patient Positioning

The patient is placed supine, head first into the scanner, and rotated slightly onto the affected side. The arm is placed down by the side and supinated. In order to bring the arm closer to the isocentre of the magnet the arm is placed on a foam pad and immobilised in a comfortable position, ensuring that the area of interest is within the sensitive range of the coil selected (Fig. 11.57).

Pulse Sequences and Scanning Planes

The spin echo pulse sequence is used and both T1- and T2-weighted images are acquired.

A localiser using a large FOV is acquired in the sagittal or coronal plane to localise the area of abnormality. From this further planes can be acquired using a smaller FOV, a slice thickness of 5–7 mm and a 256 reconstruction matrix.

Contrast Enhancement

Contrast medium is not routinely used although it can provide additional information in certain cases.

Problem Areas

Vascular artifacts can be reduced by the application of presaturation pulses placed superiorly and inferiorly. Cardiac and respiratory motion can also cause problems when the phase-encoding axis is in the *Y*-axis (left to right); a presaturation pulse placed to cover the chest will reduce these artifacts.

Wraparound (aliasing) can occur from the chest when a small FOV is employed. An antialiasing technique will minimise these artifacts.

New Improved Techniques

Fast spin echo techniques allow T2-weighted sequences to be acquired in multiple planes.

ABDOMEN

MRI of the abdomen used to be degraded by movement artifacts including respiratory and bowel movement. However, many of these artifacts have been overcome by new, faster pulse sequences. There is good contrast between the tissues which is enhanced by the peritoneal fat.

Technical Considerations

The body coil is usually used to image the abdomen and viscera, although wraparound coils are available which improve the SNR.

Patient Positioning

The patient is placed supine, head first into the scanner, and is given any instructions concerning breath-holding. This position is usually standard for imaging any of the abdominal organs.

Pulse Sequences

The spin echo pulse sequence is used to obtain T1- and T2-weighted images.

A gradient echo sequence may be useful to minimise breathing artifacts.

The STIR sequence will suppress the signal from abdominal fat, especially fat in the anterior wall, and will also reduce breathing and movement artifacts.

Fat saturation is useful in abdominal imaging, especially when imaging the pancreas which is demonstrated as a high-signal structure (because of its high water content) against the low signal of the adjacent abdominal fat. Careful adjustment of the frequency of the fat saturation pulse is essential for saturation uniformity

and good image quality.

Scanning Planes

A coronal T1-weighted sequence is acquired using a FOV of 35–45 cm, slice thickness of 7–10 mm and 256 reconstruction matrix covering from the diaphragm to the symphysis pubis.

From the appropriate coronal image a series of axial images is acquired using a FOV of 35–45 cm, slice thickness of 7–10 mm and 256 reconstruction matrix.

A STIR sequence in the appropriate plane (usually the axial plane) can be acquired to suppress the signal from abdominal fat and is useful for assessing fatty lesions in the liver. Ascites can easily be seen with the inversion recovery sequence. The combined T1 and T2 contrast obtained makes the sequence extremely sensitive to lesion detection.

Contrast Enhancement

Use of contrast will depend upon the abdominal organ being investigated and is covered in the sections on viscera below.

Problem Areas

Images of the abdomen can easily be degraded by respiratory and peristaltic motion and blood flow artifacts. There are, however, several ways of helping to overcome these in order to produce good diagnostic images.

Presaturation slabs placed anteriorly are sometimes advocated to reduce respiratory-related artifacts from the fat in the anterior abdominal wall. Superiorly and inferiorly placed presaturation bands saturate the signal from inflowing blood, preventing degradation of resultant images. Gradient motion nulling will reduce ghosting effects from blood flow and CSF pulsatile motion. Signal averaging is used to reduce ghosting artifacts which occur due to the replication of subcutaneous fat structures. Breath-hold techniques in conjunction with fast scanning sequences reduce breathing and movement artifacts and help to produce high-resolution images.

New Improved Techniques

Fast spin echo techniques allow T2-weighted sequences to be acquired in multiple planes.

When used in conjunction with fast T1 gradient echo sequences the administration of a bolus injection of i.v. contrast medium allows assessment of vascular anatomy and patency.

Phased array coils are being developed for abdominal imaging.

Magnetisation transfer is also a good method of manipulating tissue contrast and demonstrating normal and abnormal tissue. It is still being fully evaluated.

MR angiography is valuable in demonstrating the portal venous system.

Echo planar imaging allows data acquisition in milliseconds. At present the resolution is low but will improve in the future.

The Liver

The liver is a very complex organ. Its central role in the body's metabolism means it is extremely vascular, accepting blood from the abdominal organs. This fact makes the liver a prime site for metastases (Fig. 11.58) from bowel carcinomas. Although there are many imaging modalities available (e.g. ultrasound, CT, nuclear medicine), MRI can image the liver in any plane and is sensitive to the detection of liver lesions. Due to the liver's anatomical location and the lengthy imaging sequences associated with MRI, problems with respiration, bowel peristalsis and vascular motion occur.

Liver imaging techniques are designed to maximise contrast between lesion and organ and to minimise motion artifacts. Parameters change according to magnetic field strength: at high field strengths the difference in T1 values between liver and lesion is less than it is at low field strengths, while the T2 value of normal liver is shortened at high field strengths.

Haemochromatosis results in an increase in iron deposition and can affect the liver, heart, spleen, pancreas and skin. MRI shows a dramatic reduction in the normal signal intensity of the liver in patients with an iron overload as there is marked T2 shortening as a result of the deposition of haemosiderin (Fig. 11.59). Axial and coronal T1-weighted sequences will be adequate to demonstrate this. Hepatomas are sometimes found as a result of this disease and are easily visualised by MRI. MRI is helpful in the staging of haemochromatosis and after a course of therapy the liver can return to normal signal intensity.

Pulse Sequences

Spin echo T1- and T2-weighted images are well established in liver imaging. Normal liver has short T1 and T2 values, but these increase in the presence of a pathological condition. The T1-weighted sequence should be heavily T1 weighted (shortest possible TE,

i.e. 10 ms) to maximise contrast between liver and lesion. A longer TE would result in T2 effects reducing the signal from the liver and thus a reduction in contrast. The T2-weighted sequence will provide good contrast between liver and lesion because of the short T2 value of normal liver, although the long scanning times involved can lead to image degradation due to motion. Heavily T2-weighted images (TE 120–160 ms) can sometimes be useful to differentiate cavernous haemangiomas from carcinomas, because of the long T2 value of the haemangioma.

Inversion recovery sequences can be used in liver imaging. A medium TI (300–600 ms) and short TE (20–30 ms) will produce heavily T1-weighted images that provide maximum contrast between liver and lesion. A short TI (100–150 ms) and short TE (20–30 ms) will remove the signal from fat as well as providing additive T1 and T2 contrast, giving high sensitivity but low specificity (Fig. 11.58b).

The recently developed fast gradient echo scans (Turbo FLASH, Fast SPGR or TFE) make liver imaging much more practicable as they help to reduce motion artifacts and allow the acquisition of high-quality images in less than 1 s. Breath-hold sequences produce high-resolution images of the liver and can be weighted to enhance both T1 and T2 contrast. T1 weighting can be obtained using large flip angles (70°–90°) and spoiler pulses to destroy any residual transverse magnetisation. The use of a short TE time (3–5 ms) minimises T2 contrast and so makes this technique suitable for higher field strengths (Fig. 11.60).

Scanning Planes

The axial plane demonstrates the hepatic and portal veins and sometimes the hepatic artery. Axial images obtained with the patient rotated 15°–20° to the right will project ghosting away from the liver if presaturation is not available.

Coronal images help demonstrate the full extent of a lesion and show the entire course of the extrahepatic portal vein. An oblique coronal plane can be used for better demonstration of the portal vein.

The sagittal plane will demonstrate the entire length of the aorta and inferior vena cava. The relationship of the liver to the lung, diaphragm and adjacent organs can be seen in the coronal and sagittal images.

Contrast Enhancement

Oral contrast agents can be given to shorten or prolong the T1 of the bowel contents to less than or more than that of the surrounding organs.

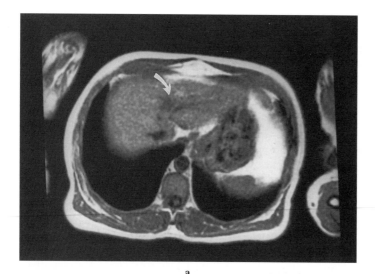

a

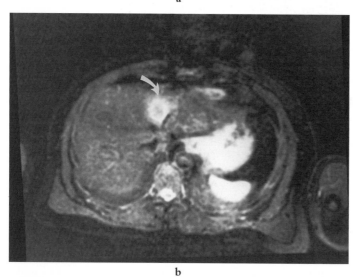

b

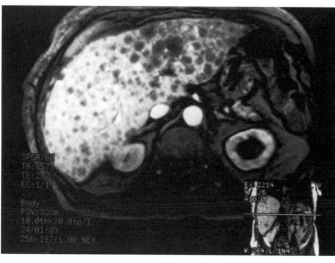

c

Fig. 11.58 a Axial T1-weighted gradient echo image (TR 40 ms, TE 12 ms, flip angle 65°) of the liver using a breath-hold technique. There is a poorly defined area of hypointensity (*arrow*) within the liver. **b** Axial STIR image (TR 2000 ms, TI 100 ms, TE 25 ms) in the same patient. The abnormal area is now hyperintense (*arrow*) and is more clearly demonstrated. This was a single metastasis. **c** Axial T1-weighted gradient echo (SPGR) image (TR 157 ms, TE 2.7 ms, flip angle 60°) of the liver using a single breath-hold technique demonstrating multiple metastases in the liver. Fat saturation has been applied. (Courtesy of IGE Medical Systems.)

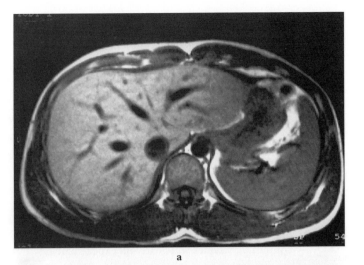

a

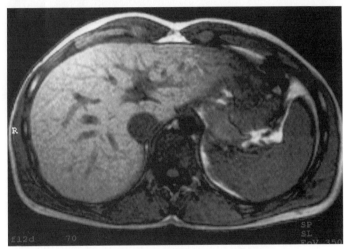

b

Fig. 11.59 **a** Axial T1-weighted SE image (TR 450 ms, TE 21 ms) of a normal liver. **b** Axial T1-weighted SE image (TR 450 ms, TE 21 ms) of a liver in a patient suffering from haemochromatosis. The deposition of iron in the liver from this condition has caused a marked T2 shortening – hence the hypointensity.

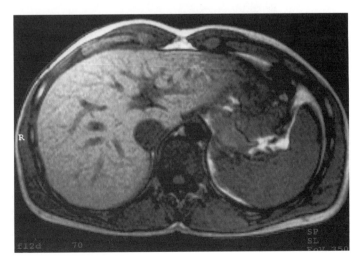

Fig. 11.60. Axial gradient echo (FLASH) T1-weighted image (TR 108 ms, TE 5 ms, flip angle 70°, acquisition time 20 s) of the liver acquired as part of a multi-slice sequence during a single breath-hold. (Courtesy of Siemens.)

Intravenous contrast medium is commonly administered and, when used in conjunction with fast gradient echo sequences, is a very sensitive method of imaging.

Research is also in progress to develop chelates which are excreted via the liver. This would allow any abnormal function to be identified. The use of intravenous microscopic iron oxide particles (MIOPs) for liver imaging is also being studied.

The Pancreas

The pancreas is not easily visualised as it has a similar T1 value to the surrounding bowel loops. Images tend to be degraded by motion artifacts and by lack of contrast between the pancreas and adjacent fat. Fast scanning multislice breath-hold techniques before and after the dynamic i.v. injection of contrast medium may provide a means of evaluating pancreatic disease. By swapping the phase- and frequency-encoding directions, ghosting from the aorta will not be superimposed onto the pancreas. Thin slices may be required to detect small lesions; otherwise 8 mm slice thickness should be adequate. The pancreas is best demonstrated in the axial plane.

Fat presaturation techniques allow good visualisation of the pancreas against its surrounding fatty tissue.

The Retroperitoneum

Disease of the retroperitoneum is best imaged in the coronal plane using a STIR sequence to suppress the signal from abdominal fat. A presaturation slab placed anteriorly will help reduce artifacts.

The Kidneys

A coronal T1-weighted sequence is acquired to demonstrate renal vascularity, the inferior vena cava and involvement of adjacent structures.

Axial T1- and T2-weighted spin echo sequences are performed with the application of presaturation slabs superior and inferior to the slices, as well as over the anterior abdominal wall. Rapid scanning techniques with bolus contrast injection and dynamic scanning will allow the detection of renal masses.

The Adrenal Glands

T1- and T2-weighted images are used to demonstrate the adrenal glands. The glands stand out against the high signal from surrounding fat on T1-weighted

sequences and these sequences are used to demonstrate their anatomy. Pathological conditions are seen on T2-weighted sequences. Fig. 11.61 demonstrates a phaeochromocytoma.

Dynamic fast scanning techniques in the coronal plane before and after the administration of a bolus contrast injection are useful in demonstrating adrenal masses.

The Spleen

The T1 and T2 values of the spleen are relatively long. This means the signal intensities of normal spleen and splenic tumours are very similar. The sensitivity of tumour detection in the spleen is low and relies on contrast techniques which are still experimental.

THE PELVIS

Problems associated with respiration, flow and bowel movement are greatly reduced in the pelvis compared with the upper abdomen.

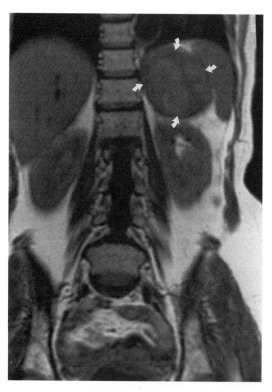

Fig. 11.61. Coronal SE T1-weighted image (TR 450 ms, TE 21 ms) of the abdomen showing a large mixed-intensity lesion in the left adrenal gland (*arrows*). This was found to be a phaeochromocytoma.

Technical Considerations

The body coil is routinely used when examining the pelvis. There are also wraparound surface coils available. Endorectal surface coils provide superbly detailed information in both the male and female pelvis.

Patient Positioning

The patient is asked not to empty their bladder for half an hour prior to the examination. The distended bladder displaces bowel loops within the pelvis allowing good visualisation of the pelvic contents and acts as a helpful landmark. Other optional patient preparations include air in the rectum, smooth muscle relaxants, a vaginal tampon and imaging in the prone position.

The patient is placed supine and feet first into the scanner.

Pulse Sequences

The spin echo pulse sequence is used and both T1- and T2-weighted images are acquired.

The STIR sequence is useful for fat suppression to assess soft tissue lesions.

Scanning Planes

T1-weighted images in all three imaging planes will give useful information. The coronal plane will show the relationship of the pelvic organs to one another and their size and position. It will also demonstrate any abnormalities on the pelvic side walls including lymph nodes. A FOV of 35–45 cm with a slice thickness of 7–10 mm and a high resolution 256 matrix are used.

The axial plane also shows the relationship of the pelvic organs and correlates with CT sections. A FOV of 35–45 cm with a slice thickness of 7–10 mm and a high resolution 256 matrix are used.

The sagittal plane is useful in assessing tumours of the bladder wall in both sexes. A FOV of 35–45 cm with a slice thickness of 7–10 mm and a high resolution 256 matrix are used.

A T2-weighted and/or a STIR sequence is performed in the appropriate plane according to clinical indications.

The Female Pelvis. The sagittal plane is essential for outlining the relative positions of the bladder, uterus and rectum (Fig. 11.62). The vaginal canal and cervix can also be seen in this plane. Three separate zones within the normal uterus may be identified. Coronal images demonstrate the broad ligaments, which is useful in identifying the ovaries and showing adnexal

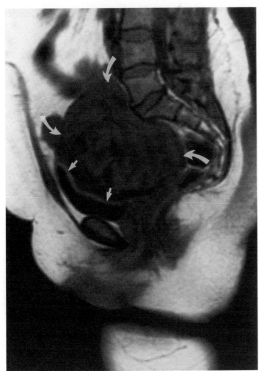

a

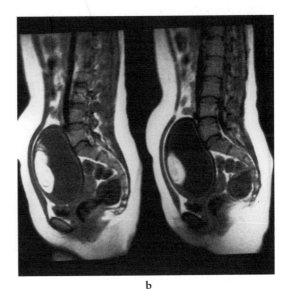

b

Fig. 11.62 a Sagittal SE T1-weighted image (TR 450 ms, TE 21 ms) of the female pelvis showing a large fibroid uterus (*curved arrows*). The bladder (*straight arrows*) is compressed by the mass. **b** Sagittal SE T1-weighted images (TR 450 ms, TE 21 ms) of the female pelvis showing a large regular mixed-intensity mass situated above the uterus and bladder that appears to occupy the whole of the pelvic cavity. This was dermoid cyst.

masses. Axial images will demonstrate the cervix, ovaries, vagina and pelvic side wall structures.

MRI is a significant advance in the staging of gynae-cological carcinoma and in follow-up after therapy.

The Male Pelvis. MRI is useful in investigating disease of the bladder and prostate gland. The sagittal plane demonstrates the prostate gland and the seminal vesi-cles which lie within the retroperitoneal fat behind the bladder. The coronal plane provides information on the integrity of the prostatic capsule and will demon-strate any pelvic lymphadenopathy. In the axial plane there is good contrast between the prostate, bladder, seminal vesicles and surrounding fat. Lymph nodes and muscles can also be readily seen.

Prostate carcinoma is the most common cancer in men and by the use of endorectal surface coils it is possible to image the prostate and associated structures (prostatic capsule, neurovascular bundle, seminal vesi-cles) with high tissue contrast in multiple planes allow-ing the staging of the local extent of the cancer. The body coil can be used but it has limited spatial resolu-tion when imaging small tumours.

An undescended testicle that cannot be palpated in the inguinal canal may be intra-abdominal, ectopic, intra-canalicular, atrophic or congenitally absent. Undescended testes may be located anywhere from the kidneys to the scrotum as well as in the superficial abdominal wall, and will be recognised best in the coronal plane using a large FOV (35–42 cm).

The testes and scrotum can also be imaged using a suitable surface coil to detect any lesions, pathology, inflammation, torsion or trauma.

Contrast Enhancement

Contrast medium is not routinely used in the pelvis but may provide additional information in some cases (Fig. 11. 63).

Problem Areas

Pelvic imaging does not usually present problems with respiratory or vascular artifacts in the way that abdomi-nal imaging does.

New Improved Techniques

The development of endoscopic receiver coils and pelvic phase array coils (Fig. 11.64) has been particu-larly valuable for examining certain small internal organs such as the prostate gland and cervix.

Fast spin echo techniques allow T2-weighted sequences to be acquired in multiple planes or the use of a 512 matrix for greater resolution. Similarly the fast inversion recovery sequences can be employed; these techniques are being further evaluated in pelvic imaging.

Obstetrics

Ultrasound, because it does not use ionising radiation, has long been the imaging modality of choice in obstetrics and has revolutionised antenatal care. However, MRI also does not use ionising radiation, it is non-invasive and it can provide images in multiple planes. Although to date there have been no adverse side effects recorded the National Radiation Protection Bureau recommends that scanning be avoided during the first trimester when rapid organo-genesis is occurring.

The patient lies supine with the legs flexed over a foam cushion, but if this is uncomfortable an oblique or decubitus position may be more tolerable.

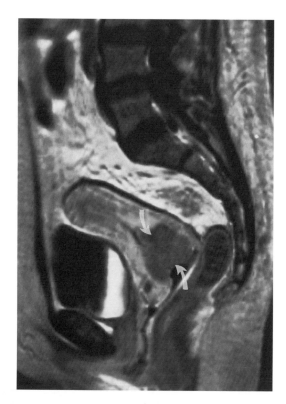

Fig. 11.63. Sagittal SE T1-weighted image (TR 700 ms, TE 15 ms) of the female pelvis after i.v. contrast medium showing nor-mal enhancement from the uterus which outlines an area of reduced enhancement in the cervix (carcinoma of the cervix: *arrows*). (Courtesy of Siemens.)

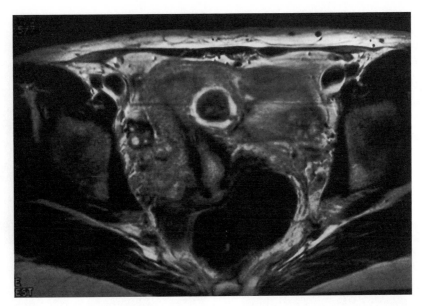

Fig. 11.64. Axial fast spin echo T2-weighted image (TR 3000 ms, TE 119 ms, 24 cm FOV, 512 reconstruction matrix) of the female pelvis using a phased array coil which demonstrates the high resolution and anatomical detail available. (Courtesy of IGE Medical Systems.)

The sagittal plane will demonstrate both the pelvic anatomy and the fetus adequately (Fig. 11.65), and axial and coronal planes will provide further information. The plane which gives the most information will depend upon the position of the fetus and the structures that are being evaluated. Fetal anatomy will obviously be delineated better as the pregnancy progresses. Movement of the fetus may degrade the images and so the shortest scanning time possible should be used.

X-ray pelvimetry, which is used to assess the adequacy of the maternal pelvis to allow the passage of the fetus, uses ionising radiation, and although pelvimetry is still performed in many centres, MRI may provide an alternative method without the use of ionising radiation. The patient is placed supine on the scanning table and sagittal T1-weighted images obtained through the pelvis. From the midline sagittal image two sets of oblique axial images are prescribed: one set parallel to and centred upon a plane from the S1/2 disc space to the superior border of the symophysis pubis and a second set parallel to a line from the sacrococcygeal junction to the inferior border of the symphysis pubis. The midline sagittal images are used to measure the anteroposterior diameter of the pelvic inlet and outlet (Fig. 11.66a) while the axial images allow the transverse (Fig. 11.66b) and interspinous diameter (Fig. 11.66c) to be measured.

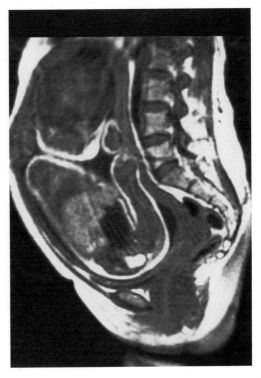

Fig. 11.65. Sagittal SE T1-weighted image (TR 450 ms, TE 21 ms) of the pelvis demonstrating a full-term fetus in the breech position.

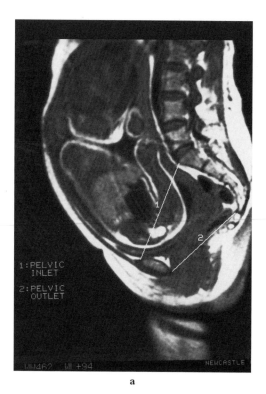

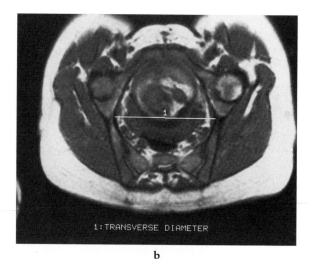

1:TRANSVERSE DIAMETER

b

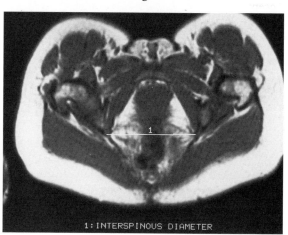

1:INTERSPINOUS DIAMETER

c

a

Fig. 11.66 a Midline sagittal SE T1-weighted image (TR 450 ms, TE 21 ms) allows measurement of pelvic inlet (*1*) and pelvic outlet (*2*) diameters. **b** Axial SE T1-weighted image (TR 450 ms, TE 21 ms) through the pelvic brim (angled from the superior portion of the symphysis to the S1/2 disc space) allows the transverse diameter to be measured as shown. **c** Axial SE T1-weighted image (TR 450 ms, TE 21 ms) from the inferior portion of the symphysis pubis to the first movable joint of the coccyx allows the interspinous diameter to be measured as shown.

BREAST IMAGING

MRI of the breast is now referred to as magnetic resonance mammography (MRM).

Mammography is the main investigation in the detection of breast carcinoma. MRI using dedicated breast coils can detect many breast conditions including cysts, scar tissue, and benign and malignant lesions with great accuracy. Lesions in the chest wall or axillary tail can be best seen on MRI. Dense fatty breasts can be a problem in mammography, but MRI using fat saturation techniques can help to visualise lesions which may be obscured by fat.

Technical Considerations

There are specially designed breast coils available to image both breasts simultaneously or one at a time.

Circular linear coils can be used to image a single breast if specially designed coils are unavailable; in the larger patient the body coil may need to be used but at the expense of loss of resolution.

Patient Positioning

The patient lies prone on the breast coil to allow the breasts to hang freely. This position will reduce the effects of respiration and give optimal image quality with the least motion artifacts. The patient is made as comfortable as possible with pads and cushions.

Pulse Sequences

Spin echo T1- and T2-weighted images are usually acquired, although gradient echo sequences have greater sensitivity especially when used in conjunction with intravenous contrast medium. Fat suppression techniques further aid in lesion detection and should be used if available. The STIR sequence can be used as an alternative method of suppressing the fat and delineating any lesions.

Scanning Planes

Thin-section sagittal and axial T1-weighted sequences are performed to cover the entire breast. A FOV is selected to cover both breasts axially (35 cm) and the single breast sagittally (25 cm) in conjunction with a 256 matrix for high resolution.

Contrast Enhancement

Recently, dynamic i.v. contrast–enhanced MRM has helped to diagnose small lesions in the breast. There tends to be delayed enhancement of benign tumours and rapid enhancement of malignant lesions. Carcinomas tend to show strong early enhancement whereas benign lesions such as fibroadenomas, cysts and scars show a slower signal increase than the carcinoma. For optimum results the dynamic i.v. contrast enhancement requires a fast scanning technique.

Problem Areas

Calcification is often an early sign of malignancy in the breast and is not readily detected by MRI, although

the use of gradient echo scans could help to overcome this.

Problems with respiration can be reduced if the patient is scanned in the prone position. Presaturation pulses can be applied to reduce artifacts from cardiac motion and swapping the phase- and frequency-encoding axes allows any residual artifacts to be directed away from the breast.

New Improved Techniques

The use of fast spin echo sequences allows T2-weighted images to be acquired in the shortest possible scanning time. Thin sections (4–6 mm) and a 256 matrix are adequate. A 512 matrix allows higher-resolution imaging. Three-dimensional spoiled gradient echo imaging can be used for the dynamic studies, providing thin slices in an acceptable acquisition time (1 minute per study).

Phase array technology has been used to develop a breast coil which allows the acquisition of extremely high-resolution images.

Breast Implants

Silicone breast implants are surgically placed for reconstruction after mastectomies or for cosmetic reasons and a method of identifying and localising leakage or ruptured implants is necessary. By using specially prepared protocols which take into account the relative

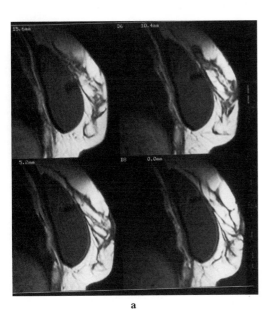
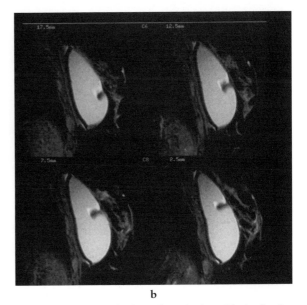

a   **b**

Fig. 11.67 a Sagittal SE T1-weighted images (TR 540 ms, TE 20 ms) in a patient with silicone breast implants. The implant has ruptured. **b** Sagittal STIR images (TR 2000 ms, TI 125 ms, TE 40 ms), by suppressing the signal from the fatty breast tissue, show the rupture more clearly. (Courtesy of Picker International Ltd.)

signal intensities of silicone, fat and water it is possible to provide diagnostic images of intact and ruptured silicone breast implants (Fig. 11.67).

The Axilla

Lesions with extensive chest wall involvement, tumours in the axilla and assessment of enlarged lymph nodes indicating metastatic spread may be readily seen using MRI.

Technical Considerations

The body coil is used in order to image both axillae simultaneously for comparison. An appropriate surface coil can be used if images of only one axilla are required.

Patient Positioning

The patient is placed supine, head first into the scanner, and made as comfortable as possible. The arms are placed by the side.

Pulse Sequences

A spin echo T1-weighted sequence is performed followed by a STIR sequence in the appropriate plane. This suppresses the signal from fat and allows good visualisation of any enlarged lymph nodes (Fig. 11.68).

Scanning Planes

A coronal localiser is acquired and axial slices prescribed from this, covering the area of interest. A FOV of 35–45 cm is used to cover both axillae in conjunction with a slice thickness of 7–10 mm and 256 reconstruction matrix. Sometimes a coronal sequence is also performed.

Contrast Enhancement

Contrast medium is not routinely administered.

Problem Areas

Motion and respiration artifacts can be reduced by ECG gating or the application of presaturation bands and/or respiratory compensation.

New Improved Techniques

Fast spin echo techniques allow T2-weighted sequences to be acquired in multiple planes or the use of a 512 reconstruction matrix for greater resolution. Similarly the fast inversion recovery sequences can be employed, possibly allowing breath-hold imaging.

CHEST AND THORAX

Mediastinum

MRI of the mediastinum gives good contrast between the high signal intensity of mediastinal fat and the low signal intensity produced by flowing blood and has proved useful in the diagnosis of a number of chest diseases located in the mediastinum, pulmonary parenchyma, pleura, hila or chest wall.

MRI is advantageous in the investigation of primary tumours or secondary spread of disease from surrounding areas such as the neck, thyroid and chest wall, and in delineating mediastinal lesions to adjacent structures. Imaging in the coronal and sagittal planes allows good visualisation of the trachea, aorta, superior vena cava and oesophagus as well as the mediastinal lymph nodes and thymus gland.

A gated spin echo or STIR sequence (useful for suppressing the signal from fat and highlighting some infiltrations) will give good results.

The Lungs

Due to the low proton density of air and the long T1 value of the lung MRI does not provide good diagnostic images. There is only a small amount of tissue present per unit volume and therefore very low signal intensity. Even when cardiac and respiratory gating are used there is still sufficient motion occurring to obscure fine detail.

CARDIOVASCULAR SYSTEM

The role of MRI in cardiac imaging is expanding rapidly and it has become useful in evaluating a wide variety of cardiac diseases. The ability to obtain images in any anatomical plane without the use of contrast media or ionising radiation makes it superior to CT.

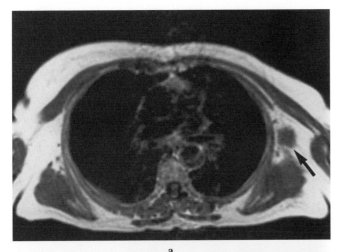

a

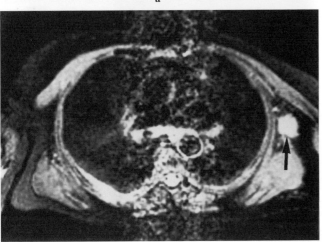

b

Fig. 11.68 **a** Axial SE T1-weighted image (TR 450 ms, TE 21 ms) showing an area of hypointensity in the region of the axilla (*arrow*). **b** Axial STIR image (TR 2000 ms, TI 100 ms, TE 25 ms) in the same patient. The signal from subcutaneous fat has been suppressed and the lesion is more readily seen (*arrow*). This represents nodal recurrence from carcinoma of the breast.

The clinical applications of MRI in the cardiovascular system are:

1. Pericardial disease (Fig. 11.69)
2. Congenital heart disease (Fig. 11.70)
3. Aortic arch disease (Fig. 11.71)
4. Acquired heart disease
5. Cardiac transplantation (Fig. 11.72)
6. Atrial and ventricular septal defects (Fig. 11.73)
7. Assessment of valve regurgitation
8. Cardiac masses (Fig. 11.74)
9. Aneurysms
10. Coarctation of the aorta (Fig. 11.75)
11. Post-operative follow-up (Fig. 11.76)

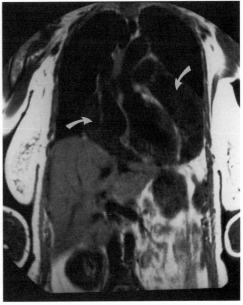

Fig. 11.69. Coronal SE T1-weighted image using ECG gating (TR 300 ms, TE 10 ms) showing a large collection in the pericardium (*arrows*). This was a haemorrhagic pericardial effusion.

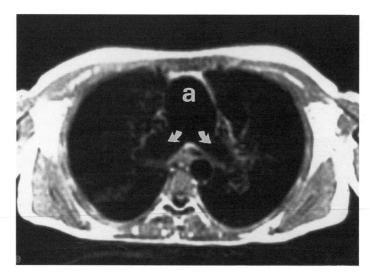

Fig. 11.70. Axial SE T1-weighted ECG gated image (TR 700 ms, TE 25 ms) of the thorax just above the heart. The left and right pulmonary arteries (*arrows*) can be seen to form one single outflow tract (*a*). This is termed truncus arteriosus.

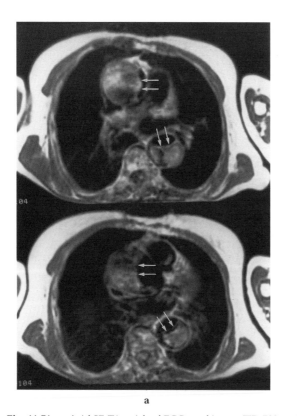

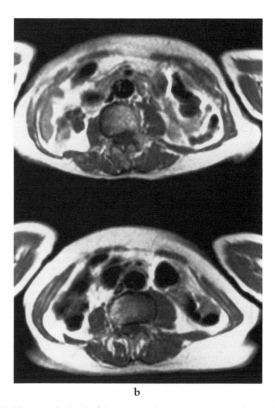

a   b

Fig. 11.71.a   Axial SE T1-weighted ECG gated images (TR 700 ms, TE 25 ms) at the level of the aortic arch in a patient with a dissected aorta. *Arrows* indicate the partition between the aortic lumen and a false channel. The high signal within the false channel is caused by stationary blood. **b** Axial SE T1-weighted ECG gated images (TR 700 ms, TE 25 ms) in the same patient. The dissection can be seen all the way down into the pelvis.

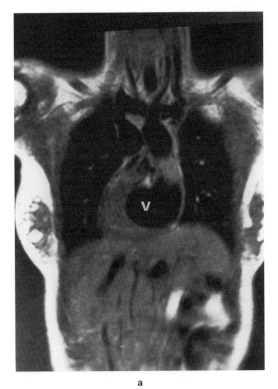

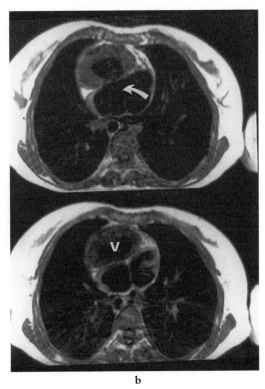

a

b

Fig. 11.72 **a** Coronal SE T1-weighted ECG gated images (TR 700 ms, TE 25 ms) showing dextrocardia with an apparent single thick-walled ventricle (*V*). **b** Axial SE T1-weighted ECG gated images (TR 700 ms, TE 25 ms) confirm the single thick-walled ventricle (*V*). Note also the defect in the septum between the two atria (*arrow*). This scan was part of a pre-operative assessment in a cardiac transplant patient.

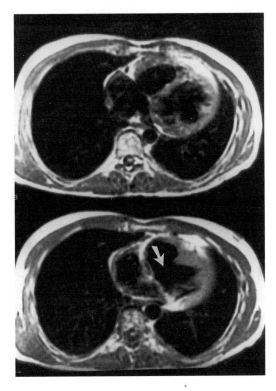

Fig. 11.73. Axial SE T1-weighted ECG gated images (TR 700 ms, TE 25 ms) showing a defect in the ventricular septum (*arrow*).

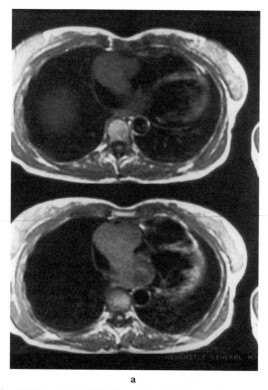
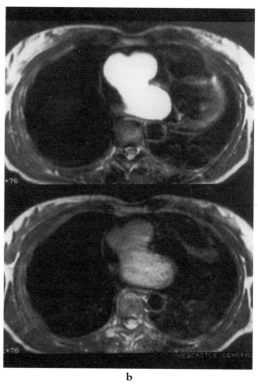

a   b

Fig. 11.74   a Axial SE T1-weighted ECG gated images (TR 700 ms, TE 25 ms) demonstrating a large mass within both atria extending through the fovea ovalis. **b** Axial SE T2-weighted ECG gated images (TR 1800 ms, TE 70 ms) in the same patient. This was diagnosed as atrial myxoma.

Technical Considerations

The body coil is used to image the heart and great vessels in the adult but it may be possible to use the head coil for small children or even the knee coil in a very small baby. Surface coils are also available for cardiac imaging.

Patient Positioning

The patient is placed supine, head first into the scanner, and is made as comfortable as possible. ECG leads are attached to the patient in the appropriate places avoiding the areas of interest.

Pulse Sequences

The spin echo pulse sequence will give good anatomical detail when used in conjunction with ECG gating. A gated STIR sequence is useful for suppressing the signal from fat and highlighting some infiltrations.

Gradient echo sequences allow a shorter TR time to be used but are not used in conjunction with ECG.

Scanning Planes

Since the heart is a very complex structure there is no standard protocol which is suitable for all eventualities. Sometimes complex angulation scans may be necessary to demonstrate the area being evaluated.

Scanning usually commences at the diaphragm and extends to the apex of the aorta. A FOV to cover the area of interest is used and a slice thickness appropriate to the size of the abnormality to be demonstrated. For example, a slice thickness of 10 mm will be adequate for large abnormalities such as large aortic aneurysms or tumours whereas a 5 mm slice thickness may be required for smaller abnormalities such as shunts. The reconstruction matrix will depend upon the FOV used but should be chosen to give the best resolution images (e.g. 256 reconstruction matrix).

The oblique sagittal plane will demonstrate the aorta and the coronal plane shows the pulmonary arteries. The long axis of the heart can be demonstrated using oblique axial scans or the oblique coronal plane. Axial images without any obliquity may be adequate in showing the long axis of the heart.

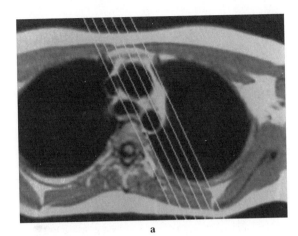

a

Fig. 11.75 **a** Axial SE T1-weighted image at the level of the aortic arch showing the reference lines for the sagittal oblique images through the aortic arch. **b** The resultant sagittal oblique SE T1-weighted ECG gated image (TR 700 ms, TE 25 ms) showing the ascending and descending thoracic aorta with coarctation (*arrow*). **c** The reference lines for the coronal oblique images to evaluate the coarctation further. **d** The resultant coronal image which again demonstrates the coarctation (*arrow*).

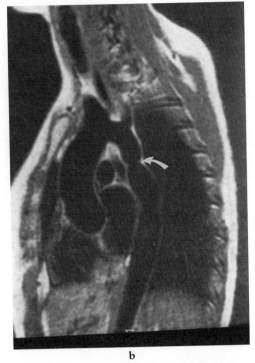

b

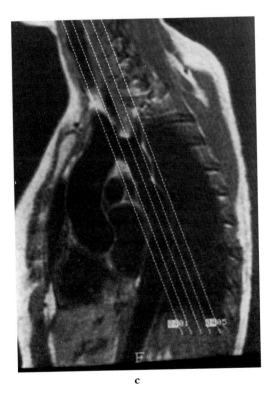

c

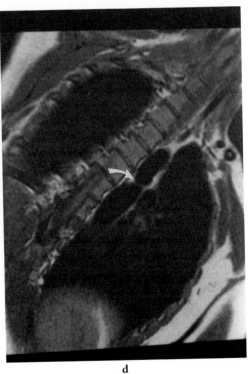

d

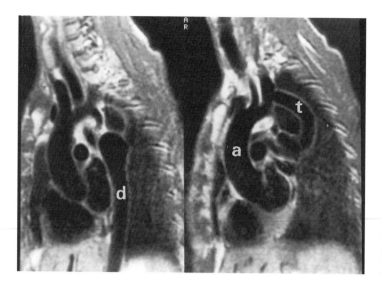

Fig. 11.76. Sagittal oblique images in a postoperative coarctation repair. A "teacup-handle" graft (*t*) has been surgically placed to redirect the blood flow around the constricted portion of the aorta. *a*, ascending aorta; *d*, descending aorta.

Contrast Enhancement

Intravenous contrast medium in conjunction with fast scanning techniques can be useful for assessing cardiac perfusion.

Problem Areas

Cardiac motion and respiration are obvious causes of artifacts in this area.

A good quality dedicated ECG system is essential and a stable ECG with an adequate R or S wave is necessary. If the electrodes contain metal they should be positioned outside the area being imaged and particular attention should be given to careful attachment of the electrodes.

The more regular the heart beat the better quality the images, but an occasional ectopic beat will not degrade the images. Frequent ectopic beats, atrial fibrillation with an irregular ventricular rhythm or sinus arrhythmia will result in serious degradation of the images.

New Improved Techniques

ECG gating using retrospective gating (which will only accept image data acquired during cardiac cycles with an R-R interval in a certain range) can improve on the images from patients with irregular heart beats, but this is not yet widely available.

Respiratory gating in combination with ECG triggering is very efficient in generating artifact-free, high-quality images in cardiac and thoracic MRI.

The development of fast scanning techniques will allow examinations to be performed more quickly and easily.

3D imaging of the heart is available which in conjunction with fast imaging techniques will give good diagnostic images in shorter acquisition times.

Flow imaging and measuring techniques are becoming available which show very clearly the flow of blood within the heart and across the valves as well as through congenital defects.

Echo planar imaging shows great potential for cardiac imaging, although the images are slightly different in appearance from conventional 2DFT images in that they tend to be strongly T2 weighted. Gradient echo planar imaging as well as spin echo planar imaging is available and can be played back in a closed loop to produce cineangiogram-like studies.

Cine MRI of the heart using ECG gating gives information on cardiac flow and function and is still being further developed.

Consecutive images, obtained through the cardiac cycle, permit assessment of myocardial dynamics. The images are used to produce a cine display when combined in a cine loop mode. Multiple slices can be imaged simultaneously with this technique.

Software is available that allows quantitative, functional analysis of the heart.

MR angiography to demonstrate the coronary arteries is still being improved (e.g. segmented breath-hold techniques).

Cardiac tagging provides an indication of heart wall motion.

High-resolution surface coil imaging, motion artifact suppression techniques, fast imaging sequences, post-processing evaluations (ejection fraction, wall thickness) and cine displays are all recent advances in cardiac MRI.

PAEDIATRIC IMAGING

Patient cooperation is essential in order to complete an MRI examination and acquire good diagnostic images. The long acquisition times can be a particular problem for children. Spending some time with the child and parents explaining what is going to happen and how the machine works may be beneficial. The parents should be encouraged to remain with the child during the examination. Sedation may be required for very young or uncooperative children.

Although the basic principles of paediatric imaging are the same as for adults there are a number of practical differences which need to be considered when performing paediatric scans.

Technical Considerations

The size of children compared with adults means that the receiver coils normally used will not be suitable. An obvious example is the use of the head coil instead of the body coil when scanning the paediatric thorax or abdomen. Receiver coils work more efficiently (increased SNR) when placed as close to the region of interest as possible. Since a child's body fills the head coil there will be a better SNR than with the body coil. Specially designed paediatric coils are now available from coil manufacturers but most MRI departments use some of the smaller coils they already possess.

Patient Positioning

The same positioning requirements that apply to adults also apply to children. Immobilisation is a key factor and compression bands or strapping are essential for all studies.

Pulse Sequences

All available pulse sequences can be used when scanning paediatric patients; the parameter selection, however, may need changing. The neonatal brain, for example, contains a larger proportion of water (92%–95%) than an adult brain. This results in a marked increase in T1 and T2 by as much as 3–4

times. Myelination is visualised best on T1-weighted images during the first 6 months of life, white matter having a lower signal intensity than grey matter. As myelination progresses there is a gradual increase in signal intensity from the white matter. From 6 months T2-weighted images will become more valuable as up to that time white matter has a higher signal intensity than grey matter on this sequence.

The inversion recovery sequence being so versatile can produce very heavily T1-weighted images and is an ideal sequence for assessing myelination. The precise parameter selection of this sequence changes with age according to the brain's water content. Table 11.4 shows how the scanning parameters of the inversion recovery sequence change with age when assessing brain development.

Scanning Planes

As with adults all three orthogonal planes are used. The area of anatomy being scanned is smaller and therefore thinner slices are used in conjunction with the largest matrix size and a suitable FOV.

Contrast Enhancement

Intravenous contrast medium is now licensed for use in paediatric patients and can be used when applicable to provide additional information. The recommended dose is 0.2 ml/kg body weight.

Problem Areas

Motion is an obvious problem in paediatric patients and the importance of the radiographer's role in gain-

Table 11.4. The changes in scanning parameters of the inversion recovery sequence according to age

Sequence	TR	TI	TE
Spin echo			
T1 dependent	720[a]		20
T2 dependent	3400[a]		120
Inversion recovery			
<40 weeks	7000[a]	2100	30
0–2 months	3800[a]	950	30
3 months–2 years	3600[a]	800	30
2 years and over	3200[a]	700	30
Short TI inversion recovery	3400[a]	150	30

Courtesy of Pennock (1992).
[a] Dependent on the number of slices.

ing the child's confidence cannot be emphasised enough. Even the most cooperative unsedated child will find it difficult to stay in the scanner for an extended period of time without moving, regardless of how well strapped and padded they are.

The age of the child being scanned will have an effect on how cooperative the child is. Neonates can often be scanned after a feed when they are naturally asleep, whereas a 2- to 4-year-old may need sedation as they are often the most uncooperative. Older children can sometimes be coaxed into being cooperative if they are allowed to see the machine and a parent remains with them. There may be a few occasions when sedation fails and a general anaesthetic is required.

The selection of pulse sequences can be tailored to reduce scanning time to a minimum. It is better to obtain a slightly lower-quality scan in a shorter time than a high-quality scan which is degraded by patient movement.

New Improved Techniques

The use of fast spin echo, fast inversion recovery and fast gradient echo sequences will help to reduce scanning times further.

Suggested Reading

Balaban RS, Ceckler TL (1992) Magnetisation transfer contrast in magnetic resonance imaging. Magnetic Resonance Quarterly 8 (2): 161–137

Barker S (1992) Magnetic resonance imaging of intracranial haemorrhage and vascular diseases. Clinical MRI 2(2):57–62

Bassett LW, Gold RH, et al. (1989) Atlas of the musculoskeletal system. Martin Dunitz, London

Beltran J (1990) MRI musculoskeletal system. Gower Medical Publishing, London

Bradley WG, Bydder G (1990) MRI atlas of the brain. Martin Dunitz, London

Brown I, Stevens JM (1992) MRI in the evaluation of white matter disease. Clinical MRI 2(2):49–55

Bydder GM, Young IR (1985) Clinical use of the partial saturation and saturation recovery sequences in MR imaging. J Comput Assist Tomogr 9:1020–1032

Cobby MJ (1992) MR imaging of meniscal and ligamentous injuries to the knee. Clinical MRI 2(4):111–120

Edelman RR, Hesselink JR (1990) Clinical magnetic resonance imaging. WB Saunders, Philadelphia

Hartnell G (1991) Cardiac magnetic resonance imaging. Clinical MRI 1(2):43–45

Hartnell G (1991) Clinical applications of cardiac MRI. Clinical MRI 1(2):51–61

Higgins CB, Silverman NH, et al. (1990) Congenital heart disease. Raven Press, New York

Horowitz AL (1991) MRI physics for radiologists, 2nd edn. Springer, Berlin Heidelberg New York

Kanal E, Shellock FG, et al. (1990) Safety considerations in MR imaging. Radiology 176:593–606

Kaut C (1992) MRI workbook for technologists. Raven Press, New York

Kean D, Smith M (1986) Magnetic resonance imaging. Williams & Wilkins, Baltimore

Keller PJ (1988) Basic principles of MR imaging (publication 7798). IGE Medical Systems, USA

Knowles RJR, Markisz JA (1988) Quality assurance and image artifacts in MRI. Little, Brown & Co., Boston

Latchaw RE (1991) MR and CT imaging of the head, neck, and spine, 2nd edn. Mosby/Year Book, St. Louis

Mink JH, Reicher MA, et al. (1987) Magnetic resonance imaging of the knee. Raven Press, New York

National Radiation Protection Bureau (1991) A broad statement on clinical magnetic resonance diagnostic procedures, vol 2, no. 1

Procknow K (1990) MR Max Plus applications guide. IGE Medical Systems, USA

Shellock FG, Curtis JS (1991) MR imaging and biomedical implants, materials and devices: an updated review. Radiology 180:541

Society of Magnetic Resonance in Medicine (1991, 1992) Abstracts.

Stark DD, Bradley WG (1991) Magnetic resonance imaging, 2nd edn. Mosby, St. Louis

Turski P (1990) Vascular MRI: applications guide. IGE Medical Systems, USA

Wehrli FW (1986) Introduction to fast-scan magnetic resonance. IGE Medical Systems, USA

Wehrli FW (1989) Advanced MR imaging techniques. IGE Medical Systems, USA

Wehrli FW, MacFall JR, Newton TH (1984) Parameters determining the appearance of NMR images. IGE Medical Systems, USA

Winkler ML, Ortendahl DA, et al. (1988) Characteristics of partial flip angle and gradient reversal MR imaging. Radiology 166:17–26

Glossary of MR Terms

acquisition time: the period required to collect the image data for a particular scanning sequence, excluding the reconstruction time.

active shimming: correction of inhomogeneities in the magnetic field by adding *shim coils*.

ADC: analogue to digital converter. Part of the interface that converts ordinary (analogue) voltages into a digital (binary) number for use by the computer.

aliasing: a phenomenon that occurs when the *field of view* is smaller than the anatomy being imaged, and which results in the anatomy outside the field of view being "folded back" into the image. Also called *wraparound artifact*.

anisotropic: non-cubic *voxels* in the context of three-dimensional imaging.

antialiasing: – see *no phase wrap*.

artifact: a signal void or intensity on the image that bears no relation to the anatomy being imaged.

attenuation: see *receive gain*.

averaging: the repeated acquisition and averaging of the same MR signal to give a better *signal-to-noise ratio*.

axial plane: a plane which divides the body into head (superior) and feet (inferior). Also referred to as the *transverse plane*.

Bo: conventional symbol used to indicate the external magnetic field strength (main magnetic field).

B1: conventional symbol for the radiofrequency magnetic field strength (90° to the main field).

bandwidth: the range within a band of frequencies.

bounce point: the point in time following an inversion pulse at which the magnetisation vector passes through zero.

CE-FAST: Contrast Enhanced Fourier Acquisition in the STeady state.

centre frequency adjustment: a procedure which allows the operator to match the system's transmit/receive frequency with the precessional frequency of the *protons* being imaged.

centre line artifact: a line that appears in the middle of the image and perpendicular to the *phase-encoding* axis. It is usually caused by instrument instabilities.

chemical shift: the difference in the frequencies of fat and water which is caused by the chemical environment. The amount of shift is proportional to the magnetic field strength.

chemical shift artifacts: artifacts caused by *chemical shift* which are parallel to the frequency direction. They appear as dark or bright bands between fat/water interfaces.

coil: single or multiple loops of wire designed either to produce a magnetic field from the current flowing through the wire or to detect a changing magnetic field by voltage induced in the wire.

computer: the computer system controls and manages the hardware in order to implement the transmission of the *radiofrequency pulses* and receive the incoming data. It processes and stores that data and allows the processed images to be viewed.

contrast (tissue): the relative difference in *signal* intensity in two adjacent tissues.

contrast agents: agents administered to alter the appearance of a tissue on an image. MR contrast agents alter the *relaxation* rates of the tissues.

contrast-to-noise ratio (CNR): the ratio of *signal* intensity differences between two areas.

coronal plane: a horizontal plane along the longitudinal axis of the body dividing it into anterior (front) and posterior (back) halves.

cross-talk: a phenomenon that occurs in multi-slice imaging when the slice profile is broadened, resulting in adjacent tissues/slices being excited.

cryogen: liquefied gas (nitrogen or helium) used as a cooling agent to sustain the low temperatures required for *superconducting magnets*.

cryostat: vacuum chambers filled with *cryogen* which maintain the constant low temperatures necessary for *superconducting magnets*.

data clipping artifact: an artifact that results from having too high a *signal* intensity, which appears on the image as a loss of *contrast* between the tissues, giving a ghost-like appearance.

decay time: the time it takes for the *signal* to decay.

dephasing: loss of *phase coherence*.

dewar: large vacuum containers that store the cryogens.

diamagnetic: a substance that will slightly decrease a magnetic field when placed within it.

diastole: the period between the end of the T-wave and the beginning of the R-wave in the cardiac cycle.

echo planar imaging (EPI): rapid *acquisition time* (60 ms) producing an image after a single excitation using a train of separately *phase-encoded* gradient echoes.

echo time (TE): time between the centre of a *radiofrequency* excitation pulse and the centre of a read-out period (echo).

echo train length (ETL): the number of echoes generated per TR in a fast *spin echo* sequence. Also known as the turbo factor.

eddy currents: electric currents induced by the changing magnetic fields in a conductor. They develop in the metal cover of the *cryostat* and other conducting structures, and if they are not compensated for they may cause image degradation.

eddy current compensation: modifications to the voltages used to operate the *gradient coils* in order to compensate for *eddy currents*.

entry phenomenon: see *flow-related enhancement*.

even echo rephasing: rephasing of moving spins on symmetric, even echoes (2, 4, 6) in *multi-echo imaging*.

excitation: the delivery of energy in the form of a *radiofrequency pulse* into a spin system.

extended matrix: see *no phase wrap*.

Faraday shield: an electrically conductive screen placed between *transmitter* and/or *receiver coils* and patient to reduce the effects of radiofrequency electric currents.

fast SPGR: fast SPoiled Gradient Recalled acquisition (IGE Medical Systems).

fat saturation technique: a frequency-specific *radiofrequency pulse* which selectively excites fat *protons* and destroys their *transverse magnetisation*, so suppressing the fat signal.

fat suppression: a method used to nullify the signal from fat, e.g. STIR, FatSat.

ferromagnetic: a substance that is attracted to the magnet. It causes large magnetic field distortions and *signal* loss.

FFE: Fast Field Echo (Philips Medical Systems).

field of view (FOV): the area (expressed in centimetres) of the anatomy being imaged.

field strength: the intensity of the static magnetic field. Low field strength systems range from 0.02 to 0.3 *tesla* and medium field strength systems from 0.3 to 1.0 tesla, while high field strength systems are more than 1.0 tesla.

filling factor: a measure of the geometrical relation-ship of the *radiofrequency coil* and the body. A high filling factor requires the size and shape of the coil to be fitted as closely as possible to the area of interest.

FISP: Fast Imaging with Steady Precession (Siemens).

FLASH: Fast Low Angled SHot (Siemens).

flip angle: the angle by which the magnetisation is rotated by the *radiofrequency pulse*.

flow artifacts: artifacts of a high signal intensity or a *signal void* depending upon the type of sequence performed.

flow compensation: method of reducing phase shifts and the associated *signal* loss. The systems gradients are used to put flowing *protons* into phase with stationary protons and to reduce *flow artifacts*. Also known as gradient motion rephasing, gradient motion artifact suppression technique or gradient motion nulling.

flow-related enhancement: increase in *signal* intensity of moving tissues (e.g. blood relative to stationary tissue). This enhancement occurs when unsaturated, fully magnetised spins replace saturated spins between *radiofrequency pulses*.

flow void: *signal* loss in rapid flow due to phase changes. Also referred to as the *washout effect*.

fold over suppression: see *no phase wrap*.

Fourier transformation (FT): a mathematical process which separates out the frequency components of a *signal* from its amplitudes as a function of time, or vice versa.

free induction decay: the *signal* which results from the stimulation of nuclei at the *Larmor frequency* by a *radiofrequency pulse*, decays at a rate determined by the *T2 relaxation time* or, more accurately, *T2* relaxation time*.

frequency encoding: a method of obtaining spatial information in one dimension. The frequency-encoding (readout) gradient is on for a period of time before and after the echo time.

fringe field: stray *magnetic field* produced by a *magnet*.

gating: a technique used to minimise *motion artifacts* by using electrocardiography or photopulse sensing to trigger the acquisition of image data.

gauss: unit of magnetic field strength. 10 000 gauss = 1 *tesla*.

ghost artifact: artifact due to spatial *misregistration* in the *phase-encoding* direction, usually from motion-induced phase shifts.

Gibbs artifact: artifact that results in non-anatomical lines parallel to the edge between tissues that have different signal intensities. Also known as a ring artifact.

Golay coils: a particular design of coil used to create *gradient magnetic fields* perpendicular to the main magnetic field.

gradient coils: three sets of coils placed within the

magnet bore in order to produce linear *gradient magnetic fields* along the three orthogonal planes when required to allow spatial location of the MR signals. The three gradients are: slice select gradient (Gx), *phase-encoding* gradient (Gy), and *frequency-encoding* gradient or *readout gradient* (Gz).

gradient echo: echo produced by a single *radiofrequency pulse* of usually <90°, which is followed by a gradient reversal. It is very sensitive to magnetic field inhomogeneities. It is useful in fast imaging and also for imaging flowing fluids such as blood or CSF.

gradient magnetic field: a magnetic field which changes in strength in a given direction. These fields are used with selective excitation to select a region for imaging and to encode the location of MR *signals* which are received from the object being imaged.

gradient motion artifact suppression technique: see *flow compensation*.

gradient motion nulling: see *flow compensation*.

gradient motion rephasing: see *flow compensation*.

gradient pulse: a briefly applied *gradient magnetic field*.

gradient ramp: the time it takes for a *gradient magnetic field* to increase from zero to the selected amplitude. Typically in the order of a few hundred microseconds to 1 millisecond.

gradient reorientation: an option which allows the operator to change the *phase-encoding* and *frequency-encoding* axes to reduce respiratory or flow-related artifacts from obscuring the area of interest.

gradient rotation: see *gradient reorientation*.

GRASS: Gradient Recalled Acquisition in the Steady State (IGE Medical Systems).

gyromagnetic ratio: see *magnetogyric ratio*.

Helmholtz coil: a pair of current-carrying coils used to produce a uniform magnetic field in the space between them.

homogeneity: uniformity of the magnetic field. This is measured in parts per million (p.p.m) and it refers to the difference in the magnetic field strength within the *bore* of the *magnet*.

image reconstruction: the process of translating raw MR data into a two-dimensional image.

inhomogeneity: lack of uniformity in a magnetic field. Expressed as parts per million (p.p.m).

interleaved slices: a technique that allows contiguous or overlapping slice locations. The slice locations that in the first data acquisition were separated by *interslice gaps*, are filled in by subsequent multislice acquisitions.

interslice gap: the space between slices.

inversion pulse: a pulse of *radiofrequency* which is sufficient to rotate the net magnetisation by 180°.

inversion recovery sequence (IR): a sequence consisting of an initial 180° *radiofrequency pulse* to invert the magnetisation followed by a 90° radiofrequency pulse.

inversion time: the time between the 180° inverting *radiofrequency pulse* and the subsequent 90° radiofrequency pulse in an *inversion recovery sequence*.

isocentre: the point at which the three gradient planes cross.

isotropic: a situation in which all three *voxel* dimensions are equal in the context of three-dimensional imaging.

K-space: the name given to an imaginary space which contains the image data prior to *Fourier transformation*. Those data consist of a matrix of points with each line corresponding to a single *phase-encoding* step and each point along that line corresponding to the point in time that the signal was collected.

laminar flow: flow which occurs in layers. The flow profile has maximum velocity flow in the centre of the vessel and the slowest flow along the vessel wall. Laminar flow usually occurs in veins and small arteries.

Larmor equation: the relationship between field strength and resonance frequency. It is expressed as $\omega_0 = \gamma Bo$, where ω_0 is the angular frequency (precessional or *Larmor frequency*), γ is the *magnetogyric ratio* and depends upon the type of nucleus being considered, and Bo is the magnetic field strength.

Larmor frequency: the frequency at which magnetic resonance can be induced in an element. Also known as the precessional or angular frequency.

longitudinal relaxation: the return of the longitudinal magnetisation to its original value after excitation.

magnet: generates a stable *magnetic field*.

magnet bore: large opening within the magnet that allows access for patients.

magnet shielding: a method of containing the stray (fringe) magnetic field from the MR system.

magnetic field: the region surrounding a magnet which produces a magnetic force on a body within it.

magnetic moment: vector quantity indicating the magnitude and direction of the torque exerted on a magnetic system, e.g. the spinning nucleus when in a *magnetic field*.

magnetic resonance (MR): absorption or emission of electromagnetic energy by nuclei in a static magnetic field after excitation by a suitable *radiofrequency pulse*. The frequency of resonance is given by the *Larmor equation*.

magnetic susceptibility: the ability of a substance to become magnetised.

magnetogyric ratio (γ): the ratio of the magnetic moment to the angular momentum of a particle. This is constant for a given nucleus.

matrix: in MR imaging, the number of pixels along the *frequency – encoding* and *phase – encoding axes*.

maximum intensity projection (MIP): a technique for producing multiple projection images from a volume of image data (three-dimensional volume or two-dimensional stack of slices) in which the volume is processed along a selected angle. The *pixel* with the highest signal intensity is projected onto a two-dimensional image.

Maxwell pair: a coil design used to create *gradient magnetic fields* along the direction of the main magnetic field.

misregistration: artifact caused by motion or *aliasing* which results from the incorrect spatial location of the signal.

motion artifact: artifact caused by patient movement. This can be voluntary or involuntary (e.g. peristalsis, respiration).

MP-RAGE: Magnetisation Prepared RApid Gradient Echo (Siemens).

multi-echo imaging: imaging using a train of echoes following a single *radiofrequency pulse*.

multi-slice imaging: a technique for increasing the number of slices that can be acquired in a certain time. Slices which are not necessarily adjacent are imaged while waiting for relaxation of the first slice.

no phase wrap: an option that minimises *aliasing* in the *phase-encoding* direction when the anatomy being imaged is larger than the *field of view*.

nucleon: the generic name for protons and neutrons.

number of excitations (NEX): see *number of signal averages*.

number of signal averages (NSA): the number of times a *pulse sequence* is repeated in a given acquisition.

Nyquist theory: a theory that states that the periodic signals (frequencies) must be sampled at least 3 times per cycle and, in order to characterise the *signal*, at twice the highest frequency. If the signal is not sampled enough times then it is interpreted as a lower frequency and *misregistration* occurs.

oblique plane: a plane which is non-orthogonal.

odd-echo dephasing: signal loss which occurs on the first and subsequent odd echoes due to in-plane moving spins.

offcentre FOV: A *field of view* that is not centred at the *isocentre*.

orthogonal plane: anatomical planes of reference perpendicular to one another: axial, sagittal and coronal planes.

out-of-phase image: see *phase difference image*.

oversampling: a method for eliminating aliasing by acquiring extra *frequency-encoding* samples or oversampling along the *phase-encoding* direction and increasing the *field of view*. See *no phase wrap*.

paramagnetic: a substance which causes a slight increase in the magnetic field when placed within it.

partial saturation: a technique of applying repeated 90° *radiofrequency pulses* with *TR* times less than or equal to the *T1 relaxation time* of the tissues.

passive shimming: the correction of inhomogeneities in the magnetic field by adding small pieces of steel.

permanent magnet: a magnet the permanent field of which originates from permanently magnetised material. Its *fringe fields* are minimal.

phantom: an artificial object of known properties and dimensions used to test various aspects of the MR equipment.

phase coherence: signals of the same or similar frequencies that have the same phase. Loss of phase coherence of the spins results in a decrease in *transverse magnetisation* and therefore a decrease in the MR *signal*.

phase contrast angiography: two-dimensional or three-dimensional imaging technique which relies on velocity-induced phase shifts to distinguish flowing blood from stationary tissue. Two or more acquisitions with opposite polarity of the bipolar flow encoding gradients are subtracted to produce an image of the vessels.

phase difference image: an image in which signal cancellation occurs in *voxels* containing both fat and water *protons* owing to *chemical shift* effects.

phase encoding: part of the process of locating the MR *signal* by sequentially changing the *gradient magnetic field* strength by a known amount.

phase-encoding steps: the number of times that the data is sampled in the *phase-encoding* direction (directly related to overall *acquisition time*).

phase image: an image computed from the real and imaginary images in which the *pixel* brightness is proportional to the amount of phase shift within the *voxel*.

photopulse sensing: method of monitoring a patient's pulse using a light source attached to the patient's finger.

pixel: the smallest part of a digital image display. Also referred to as the picture element.

plug flow: flow in which all components are moving at the same velocity.

precession: gyration of the axis of a spinning body which traces out a cone.

precessional frequency: see *Larmor frequency*.

presaturation: a method for reducing *flow artifacts* or *motion artifacts* by applying extra *radiofrequency pulses* to specified areas in order to eliminate *signal* from those areas.

prone: a position in which the patient lies face down on the scanning table (cf. *supine*).

proton: a positively charged nucleon.

proton density: the tissue concentration of mobile hydrogen atoms.

proton density weighted: pulse sequences with parameters set to bring out the differences in the proton densities of the tissues being scanned.

PSIF: FISP reversed (Siemens).

pulse programmer: a computer system which controls the timing, shape and strength of the *radiofrequency pulse* and gradient pulses.

pulse sequence: a train of precisely timed *radiofrequency pulses* used in conjunction with *gradient magnetic fields* to excite the tissue and produce MR *signals*.

quadrature coil: *radiofrequency coil* which can detect two phases of precessing magnetisation. It results in an increase in the *signal-to-noise ratio*, theoretically by as much as 40%, and a reduction in power deposition by as much as 50%.

quenching: sudden loss of superconductivity which causes rapid evaporation of the *cryogens*.

radiofrequency (RF): the frequency of electromagnetic radiation.

radiofrequency bandwidth: the range of frequencies contained within a *radiofrequency pulse*.

radiofrequency coil: a current-carrying coil used to transmit *radiofrequency pulses* (*transmitter coil*) or to detect the MR *signal* (*receiver coil*).

radiofrequency pulse (RF): a brief burst of *radiofrequency* at the *Larmor frequency* which is delivered to the object being scanned.

radiofrequency shield: a construction of a conductive material (usually aluminium or copper) used to reduce surrounding *radiofrequency* noise within the *bandwidth* of the MR *signal* of interest.

ramp time: the time it takes for the field strength of a *superconducting magnet* to increase from zero to the operating field strength.

readout gradient: the gradient first applied when an MR *signal* is collected that is used for *frequency encoding*.

readout period: see *sampling time*.

receive gain: amplification factor of the received MR *signal* that ensures it falls within the dynamic range of the ADC.

receiver bandwidth: the range of frequencies which can be received and properly digitised.

receiver coil: coil or antenna positioned within the *magnet bore* to detect the MR *signal*.

reconstruction: the process of creating a displayable image from the scan data.

reconstruction time: the time it takes from the start of *reconstruction* to the end of reconstruction.

rectangular field of view: a field of view in which the acquisition matrices are asymmetrical (e.g. 192 × 256).

refocusing: see *spin echo*.

region of interest (ROI): operator-defined area to be statistically analysed.

relaxation: the emission of energy which causes the nuclei to go from a high-energy state back to a low-energy state.

rephasing gradient: a *gradient magnetic field* applied after the slice selective pulse to correct for the unwanted phase errors due to the gradient. This correction rephases the spins and forms an echo.

repetition time: see *TR*.

resistive magnet: an electromagnet which requires continual electrical current to maintain its magnetic field.

respiratory compensation: a modification of *phase encoding* to minimise *ghost artifacts* caused by respiratory motion.

ring artifact: see *Gibbs artifact*.

rise time: see *gradient ramp*.

R-R interval: the length of one cardiac cycle from one R-wave to the next.

R-wave: the part of the cardiac QRS complex which usually has the greatest amplitude. There is one R-wave per heart beat.

saddle coil: a *radiofrequency coil* used with solenoidal-type *superconducting magnets*.

sagittal plane: a longitudinal plane dividing the right side of the body from the left.

sampling interval: the time used to measure the *signal* for each data point during the *sampling time*.

sampling time: The time period during which an echo is collected. Also known as the readout period.

saturated protons: protons which have experienced a 90° *radiofrequency pulse* in a different slice. Hence when they flow into the selected slice they give an intermediate signal as they have not fully relaxed since their excitation.

saturation: a state when equal numbers of spins are aligned parallel and antiparallel to the magnetic field, resulting in no net magnetisation.

saturation pulse: see *presaturation*.

saturation recovery sequence (SR): a pulse sequence using repeated 90° *radiofrequency pulses* with a *TR* greater than the *T1 relaxation time* of the tissues.

selective excitation: the use of a *radiofrequency pulse* of narrow *bandwidth* which excites a volume of material in the presence of a *gradient magnetic field*.

selective pulses: *radiofrequency pulses* of a narrow *bandwidth* having a range of frequencies which correspond to the *Larmor frequencies* of the nuclei in the chosen slice (slice selective).

sequence controller: see *pulse programmer*.

shim coils: smaller magnet coils contained within the main magnet bore to maintain as homogeneous a magnetic field as possible. In addition iron plates or rods can be placed inside and outside the magnet to improve homogeneity further.

shimming: a process of improving the homogeneity of the static magnetic field. See *active shimming* and *passive shimming*.

signal: the MR signal is the electromagnetic energy released by the hydrogen nuclei in the tissues being scanned.

signal averaging: a method for improving the *signal-to-noise ratio* by using multiple excitatory *radiofrequency pulses* and taking the average of the resultant signals.

signal-to-noise ratio (SNR or S/N): a measure of the graininess of an image.

signal void: an area which contains no signal.

slice: the effective physical extent of the "planar" region being imaged, *or* location within selected anatomy.

slice gap: the distance between the centres of adjacent slices. A large slice gap is required when the slice profile is not rectangular, to prevent *cross-talk*.

slice select gradient: the gradient associated with the system's scanning direction. Usually corresponds to the direction of the scanning range.

slice selective excitation: the excitation of *protons* in one slice acquired by applying a *gradient magnetic field* (Gz) and a slice selective *radiofrequency pulse*.

slice thickness: the thickness of the imaging slice.

solenoid coil: a *radiofrequency coil* consisting of wire wrapped around a cylinder that is used in conjunction with *permanent magnet* or *resistive magnet* systems which have a vertical static field design.

spatial resolution: the dimensions of the *voxels* used in the acquisition *matrix*. It is the distance between two points at which the points can be distinguished as being separate and distinct.

spin density weighted: another name for proton density weighted.

spin echo: a pulse sequence comprising a 90° *radiofrequency pulse* followed by a 180° refocusing *radiofrequency pulse* (at TE/2) which generates an MR signal (at *TE*) directly proportional to the *T2* of the tissues.

spin–lattice relaxation times: also known as longitudinal relaxation. See *T1 relaxation time*.

spin–spin relaxation times: also known as tranverse relaxation. See *T2 relaxation time*.

spin system: the precessing nucleus of a nuclear magnetic isotope.

spoiler gradients: *a gradient magnetic field* used to eliminate residual signal by *dephasing* the spins.

spoiler pulse: the application of a *radiofrequency pulse* to eliminate *transverse magnetisation*.

steady state free precession (SSFP): multiple *radiofrequency pulses* applied rapidly and repeatedly with short intervals between them (IGE Medical Systems).

STIR: Short Tan Inversion Recovery. *Inversion recovery sequence* using a short *inversion time* to minimise the signal from fat.

superconducting magnet: a magnet the magnetic field of which originates from current flowing through a *superconductor*.

superconductor: a material which loses all electrical resistance below a critical temperature.

superparamagnetic: a substance with a large positive magnetic susceptibility.

supine: a position in which the patient lies face up on the scanning table (cf. *prone*).

surface coil: a radiofrequency *receiver coil* placed over the area of interest.

swap phase and frequency: see *gradient reorientation*

systole: the period between the R-wave and the end of the T-wave in the cardiac cycle.

T1 FFE: T1-weighted Fast Field Echo (Philips Medical Systems).

T1, inversion time: the time between the centre of the first (180°) inverting pulse and the beginning of the second (90°) refocusing pulse in an *inversion recovery sequence*.

T1 relaxation time: the time constant for the spins to regain longitudinal magnetisation after the application of a *radiofrequency pulse*.

T1-weighted: *pulse sequences* with parameters set to bring out the difference in the *T1 relaxation times* of different tissues.

T2 decay: the loss of phase coherence between spins in the magnetic field after the application of a *radiofrequency pulse*. Also known as transverse relaxation.

T2 FFE: T2-weighted Fast Field Echo (Philips Medical Systems).

T2 relaxation time: the time constant for loss of *phase coherence* among the spins which is caused by interactions between the spins in a uniform magnetic field and results in loss of *transverse magnetisation*.

T2-weighted: *pulse sequences* with parameters set to bring out the difference in the *T2 relaxation times* of different tissues.

T2★ relaxation time: the time constant for loss of *transverse magnetisation* and MR *signal* due to T2 and local field inhomogeneities.

TE, echo time: the time interval from the first *radiofrequency pulse* of a pulse sequence to the middle of a *spin echo* or a *gradient echo*.

tesla: SI unit of a magnetic field. 1 tesla = 10 000 gauss.

TFE: Turbo Field Echo (Philips Medical Systems).

three-dimensional Fourier transformation (3DFT): a method in which a thick slice of tissue is excited and *phase encoding* takes place in both the slice select and phase – encoding directions. This allows thin contiguous slices to be acquired; the *signal-to-noise ratio* is improved as signal from the entire slab is repeatedly sampled.

time of flight (TOF): see *flow-related enhancement*.

tip angle: see *flip angle*.

torque: a force that produces rotation.

TR, repetition time: the time interval from the beginning of one pulse sequence to the beginning of the next pulse sequence.

transmitter/receiver coils: *radiofrequency coils* placed inside the *gradient coils*. The radiofrequency transmitter coil converts electrical power into an oscillating magnetic field in order to excite the nuclei of the different tissues being imaged. A radiofrequency receiver coil detects the small signals produced from these tissues. This signal is then amplified and sent to the receiver.

transverse magnetisation: the part of the magnetisation vector which is perpendicular to the static magnetic field *Bo*. The MR *signal* can be detected when the transverse magnetisation precesses at the *Larmor frequency*.

transverse plane: see *axial plane*.

transverse relaxation: see *T2 decay*.

tuning: a process that allows for the calculation of the amount of *radiofrequency* power required to produce the desired *flip angles*. It is also the process of adjusting the resonant frequency of the system to the frequency of the subject being imaged, i.e., the *Larmor frequency*.

turbo factor: see *echo train length*.

turbo FLASH: turbo Fast Low Angled SHot (Siemens).

turbulence: chaotic flow pattern that usually occurs with rapid flow through a stenosis and produces signal loss due to phase dispersion.

two-dimensional Fourier transformation (2DFT): a technique used to reconstruct raw image data into two-dimensional images. The images are composed of *pixels* the brightness of which is proportional to the intensity of the MR *signal*.

unsaturated spins: spins exhibited by nuclei which have not been exposed to a *radiofrequency pulse*.

vector: a quantity that has both magnitude and direction. It is represented by an arrow, the length of which is proportional to the magnitude while the arrowhead indicates its direction.

velocity: displacement per unit time. It is measured in centimetres per second.

view: a row in a raw data set.

volume imaging: a technique in which the signal is collected from an entire volume instead of individual slices. It allows reconstruction of very thin slices and enhances the *signal-to-noise ratio*.

vortex flow: flow in localised, slowly swirling or stagnant blood which can occur as a result of a sudden deceleration distal to an area of stenosis.

voxel: a three-dimensional area of an imaged object.

washout effect: see *flow void*.

wraparound artifact: see *aliasing*.

Index